THE DRAGON I COULDN'T SLAY

True Confessions of a Caregiver

NANCY TRAIL

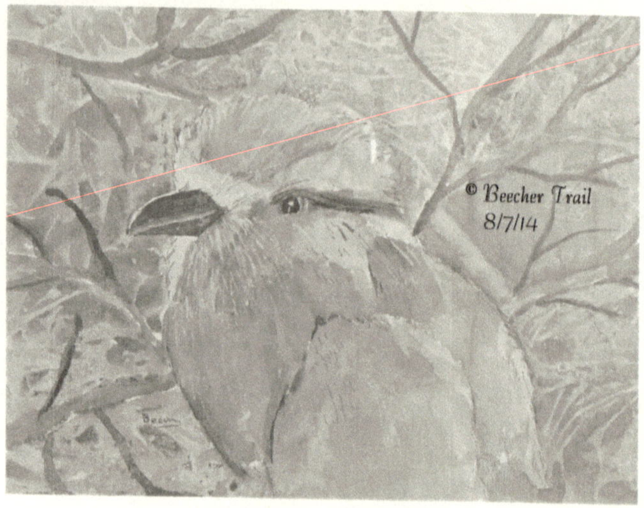

"Colorful Bird"
Watercolor by Beecher Trail - 2014
The many shades of FTD

The Dragon I Couldn't Slay ~ True Confessions of a Caregiver

Copyright © 2022 by Nancy Trail.

All the stories in this book are true.

FIRST EDITION

ISBN-979-8-88757-793-7 Paperback

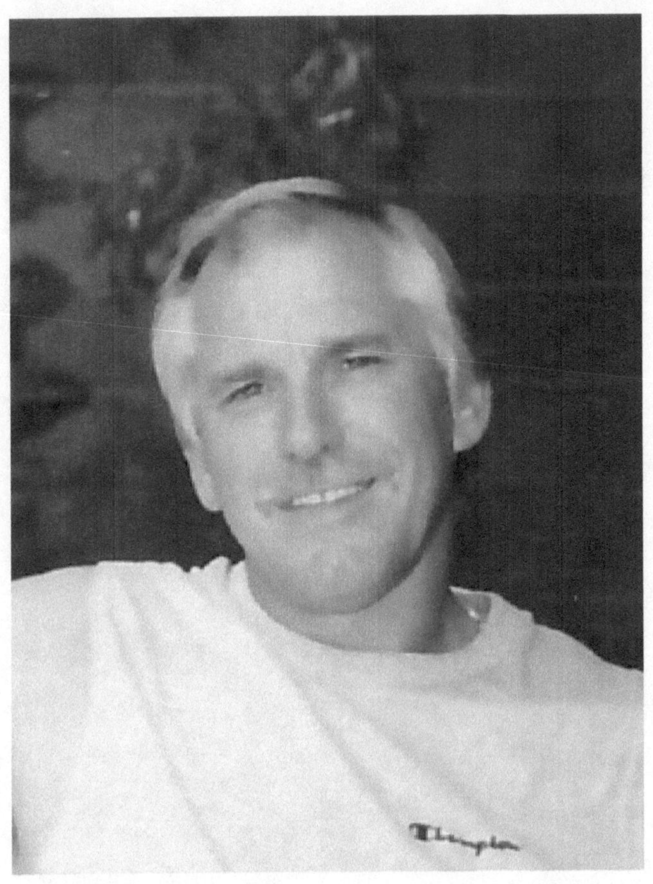

This book is dedicated to my loving husband, Beecher, who lost his life to the devastating disease called Frontotemporal Degeneration, also called Frontotemporal Dementia (FTD), and to all the caregivers who have walked my journey or have a loved one who has just been diagnosed.

October 2, 1954–October 21, 2016

"I love you to the Beech and back"

CONTENTS

FOREWORD

Life throws us challenges every now and then. Some will be experienced by most, if not all of us: marriage and sometimes divorce, birth of a child, passing of a loved one, job loss, moving, and others. Most such events, difficult as they may be, are just that: events. They are punctual and limited in time. Although they will leave their mark and contribute to shaping our character and attitudes, they should quickly become part of our past, our experience.

Some life challenges are different though. Many of you may see a loved one, a parent or a life partner, experience cognitive decline and ultimately dementia. The increased reliance on you can be slow, gradual, and prolonged. You will ultimately take on the role of caregiver. The importance and need for your support, and even your physical and emotional presence, sometimes welcomed, sometimes not, is a long-term affair. The challenges are ever present, but also fluid, changing, and will follow you through the course of your loved one's illness, and then beyond.

Fewer of us will experience caregiving for a loved one with FTD. In this rare and frequently unrecognized disorder, there will ultimately be cognitive decline and dependence, but there is first, often years before, a subtle and relentless shift in personality and behavior that can often blindside you. As your loved one's character crumbles, and their interactions with you and others lead to the dissolution of those connections so crucial to friendship, intimacy, and partnership, it may be difficult to see them as suffering or even in need. It may be difficult to truly feel connected, motivated, or even able to care.

Well, not for Nancy and Beecher. Their love affair was so deep, and so strong. Nancy remained at Beecher's side through thick and thin. She grew, perhaps initially unwittingly, to become Beecher's most ardent and vocal advocate, arguably at times despite him. She relentlessly pursued an explanation for what was happening, what was going wrong. Years later, an answer and diagnosis at hand, the process for her was still just beginning.

In her book, *The Dragon I Couldn't Slay,* Nancy exposes for us their journey. Her narrative is personal and intimate. It is also deeply spiritual and at times mystical. Sometimes raw, and ever present, her inner dialog struggles to comprehend and reconcile the complex and conflicting feelings of loss, guilt, anger, responsibility, admiration, devastation, mixed with the desire to move forward and for it to all be done with.

While FTD patients live in the moment, often without much concern for the past or the future, Nancy pulls the threads of their evolving experiences together. Beecher, unbeknownst to him, also plays an important role. The unwavering love he gave his friends and family before his illness secured a strong collective memory of him. Nancy serves as the medium that revitalizes his character and his love of life, neither of which she would allow this devastating illness to erase.

Although there may be formal means of cognitively preparing for the task of caring for someone with FTD, this book will bring you in close, emotionally, and personally. Nancy's thoughts, feelings, and angst, as well as her resourcefulness and perseverance, are on full display. Yes, the disease takes its toll on loved ones, but when it's all said and done, the caregiver can and must heal (to quote Nancy), and she shows us *her way.*

Gabriel Léger, MD
Neurologist

PREFACE

Being a caregiver is never an easy job. It's a daunting task caring for a loved one with dementia. Looking after someone with Frontotemporal Degeneration (FTD), a degenerative neurological disease, which the average person has never heard of, leaves many caregivers feeling isolated and lost in their journey.

In her book, *The Dragon I Couldn't Slay*, Nancy Trail shares her eight-year journey caring for her husband, Beecher. It is important reading, giving insight into caregiving for an FTD patient who, over time, will change in behavior, speech, and mobility. Nancy also shares pertinent information from the many professionals she met along the way.

It is a raw, honest depiction of her day-to-day struggles Nancy confronted. The account of her journey is interspersed with the humor one needs to have in many of the situations that occur.

Read how being thrown into a crisis, Nancy found the courage to be her husband's advocate, developed the resolve to search out whatever was needed to keep Beecher participating in life and discovered a way to begin her new reality in life.

Lisa Radin - Former Caregiver and Co-Author,
What if It's Not Alzheimer's? A Caregiver's Guide to Dementia

INTRODUCTION

As of this printing, it's been six years since the love of my life passed away, but it seems like yesterday as I write this book. When I started journaling and then writing this book, I had no idea how much work it was going to be. But I knew in my heart, it had to be done. For me, it had to be done so I could start moving forward. When you lose someone, you love so much, you want to make sure you give them due justice. My husband had no idea of what was happening to him or at least he didn't appear to. I thought I would have had this book published a long time ago. A weird thing happens though; you get caught up in the daily things to do, and the book just got put on the back burner.

First, I had four years of picture albums including a memorial book of him that I had neglected due to his illness. I knew if I didn't finish them right away, they would never get done.

I also had to prepare a book of Beecher's poetry. His handwritten poems had to be typed and put in chronological order to get ready to send to Shutterfly to publish. Once I got on a roll, it actually went pretty fast but it was another thing I needed to get done to honor him. I knew if I let more time lapse, I would never go back to it. Grief is hard to get through and I don't know if I ever will, but he was such a big part of my life and his words meant a lot to me. I wanted to share them with my family.

Someone once told me that grief is just love. It's all the love you want to give but cannot. All of that unspent love gathers up in the corners of your eyes, the lump in your throat, and in the hollow part of your chest. Grief is just love with no place to go.

I think this defines it for me. I made extra copies of Beecher's book of poems and gave them to my daughters. They were elated to have his poetry collection, including a poem that he had written for each of them.

Next, I needed to organize all of his watercolor pictures and put them in a portfolio. I wanted to save them in a safe place for me as well as my loved ones. I already had my favorite paintings of his hanging in my home, but I hung many more after he passed.

My fourth task was to edit and prepare this book, which is my last task to honor him and to hopefully help others in their journey through this devastating disease. When I started this journal, it was for my own sanity to help get me through the day, but now that I have finished it, I realize it's more of a self-help book with words of wisdom, truth, honesty, encouragement, feelings of despair and frustration. In many ways it is a diary as well as the journal of my journey through the many faces of FTD.

I've included some medical information pertinent to FTD as well as valuable resources that I stumbled upon (why create the wheel?), and references that I think will help others in their journey. Reading other peoples' journey helps you feel that you are not alone. It is a very lonely journey since so few have heard of the disease nor experienced it.

I want you to know that I feel empathy for you, as I have walked in your shoes. Sometimes we feel like no one understands our loss and what we've been through when we try to explain what FTD does to us, and how long it takes to heal. The grief is overwhelming as we not only experience grief when they are gone but we have experienced so much more during the journey as our loved ones slowly disappear from us. Unlike Alzheimer's that steals ones memory, **FTD steals who** we are. That is the tragedy of FTD. The person that we once knew is now replaced with a person who has lost their personality, their behavior and manners change and they are no longer recognizable to us.

The FTD wound is torn into many different directions and is full of infection. Our wounds can't heal until the infection is gone, and since it is such a nasty wound, it takes longer for us to heal. Sometimes the only people who really understand and who you can talk to are your doctor, and a few people you know who won't judge you or someone who has been through it as well. I pray for all of you that are going through it or have been through it. And I sincerely pray that a cure will come so no one ever has to experience this devastating disease.

Some of my daily posts include "our life in general" and may seem un-noteworthy to some but they are included so I have all my memories in one place. I feel a real sense of relief as I write this that I can now move forward onto the next stage of my life and learn to continue to let go as I experience new adventures without Beecher.

"There are four kinds of people in the world. Those who have been caregivers. Those who currently are caregivers. Those who will be caregivers, and those who will need caregivers. "
Rosalynn Carter – Former First Lady
(Credit and thanks to Rosalynn Carter)
I Married an Alien or an Addict? as told by a "Normie"

"Alien"

A creature from another planet other than Earth or from another universe.

"Addict"

Someone who is addicted to drugs, alcohol, sex or gambling. It is also called substance abuse and is quite often compulsive, physiological and sometimes referred to as a brain disorder.

"Normie"

A non-addict or someone who doesn't use alcohol or drugs and does not have any other addictions and is considered a normal person.

AUTHOR'S NOTE

To everyone reading this book,

Partway through my journey with FTD, I started writing in a journal to ease some of my frustrations of dealing with the many faces of FTD. I realized I wasn't the only one suffering through this battle. I was not alone and my feelings of guilt were quite normal, but I did not feel so at the time. It was through trial and error that I handled each situation on a daily basis. I later realized that other people must have felt the same way as I did. I never thought that I could disclose some of my feelings like I did in this book, but I realized it was necessary to get the message out, "that it's okay to feel what you are feeling."

Nobody taught us how to relate to our loved ones or understand this disease. With all the books on childcare that have been published over the years, parents have realized that the information doesn't always hold true for each child. At the time it seems like you are raising all of them the same way and yet each and every one turns out differently. And each person afflicted with FTD is just as different as each child. The difference between child rearing and FTD is that our children grow up or forward, but our loved ones afflicted with FTD move backward. This is the most heart-breaking part of FTD. It's like going back in time, and there is no rhyme or reason for it. It just is what it is. The outcome is always death. I pray that this book about FTD helps others deal with what I call "The Dragon I Couldn't Slay." ~True Confessions of a Caregiver~

I read somewhere that the brain turns into a carnival when we tell our stories. Lights switch on in our heads and neurons fire more rapidly. Oxytocin, a natural feel-good hormone, is released in large amounts, whether the story is happy or sad. Through telling our stories, we are reimagining ourselves. It happens even more when we hear other people's stories. Through stories we all survive. I hope I will bring those feel-good feelings to you even though my story is a sad one.

To Beecher,

Missing you is a heartache that never seems to go away. My life has gone on without you, but it will never be the same. I am fortunate to have your many poems, the numerous photos, the watercolors and all the memories you gave all of us throughout our marriage and this journey. Thank you for the lessons. I now know the meaning of the statement, "I am not defined." Defining who I am is about removing the labels and expectations others including myself, placed on me and recognizing that my past does not define me or my future.

CHAPTER 1

2010-2011—THE BEGINNING

"WHERE DID MY HUSBAND GO?"

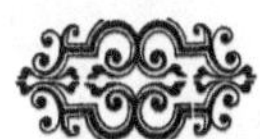

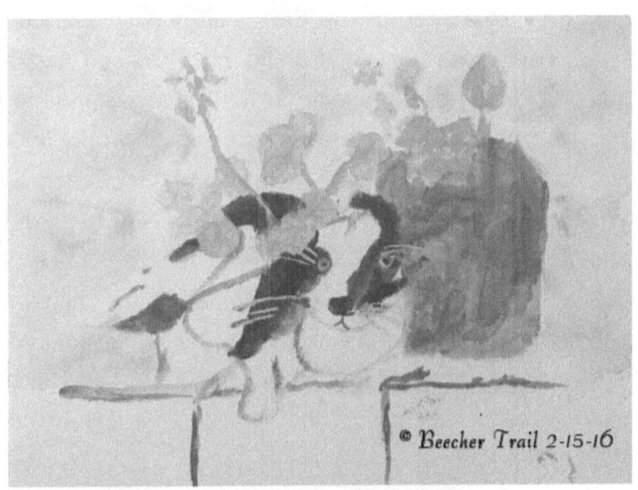

"Rabbit in Hiding"
Watercolor by Beecher Trail
"A rabbit represents abundance, comfort, vulnerability,
sentiment, desire, and the seasons with changes
in Mother Earth, especially springtime"

I t was in the spring of 2011 when I woke up one morning and found a strange man in my bed! Who was he and how did he get here? Oh my gosh, I thought, what should I do? He kind of looked like my husband, but he didn't act like my husband. His eyes were kind of glassy and he had a blank stare on his face. And he couldn't talk very good. As I backed away from him, I asked him how he got here. He shrugged his shoulders, and quietly told me he didn't know either. I thought I must be having a nightmare, but just in case I wasn't, I ran out of the house away from this intruder. When I reached the end of the street, I realized I was in my pajamas and then the reality set in. This was real and a living nightmare had just begun!

Prior to this realization, life in early 2010 and 2011 seemed somewhat normal, like a soft little bunny rabbit in hiding. Sometime during this two-year period, I started noticing some unusual changes in my husband Beecher. He wasn't always the social person he used to be. He was always playing with his iPhone and his iPad and a game called Angry Birds. My daughters and some of his friends seemed to notice as well and we just thought he was under stress with work. In November 2011, he got into two car accidents within six days of each other. Both were with his company truck at the same location getting on the freeway. Not only did we have to pay $1000 each time for the deductible, but his company took away his work truck and he had to use his own vehicle. Since he was in Sales, he put a lot of mileage on his car and had to get a new car. This meant higher insurance and bigger car payments. I started doing some craft shows selling my homemade foot jewelry to help out with the higher bills.

Backtrack to the beginning of our relationship–1988

As a young man, Beecher or "Beech" (as he was mostly called) was full of life and ambition. The sky was the limit for all the things he wanted to do and the places he wanted to go. Even though he was insecure in his past relationships (seeing how his birth mother had been married thirteen times), he wanted to beat the odds and be the one-in-a million who was successful. He had been married once before and I had been married twice but we hit it off right away. Both of our mothers' name were Etta; mine was Etta Mae and his was Etta Naomi. We both had young daughters about the same age. My youngest was eleven and his stepdaughter was ten. I also had older children 21 and 24. I was eight years older than him. I think I was a Cougar before the term was even invented! I had been through some rocky relationships after my last divorce and I was ready to settle down.

The night we met in late November 1988, I went to meet a high school friend for drinks. She had just met him that day and invited him to join us. After several hours of getting to know him, he offered to follow me home since I had had a few drinks. Come to find out we lived in the same apartment building, two buildings away. Destiny! I was sure I had found my soul mate! A week later we started dating and that's where my journey started. How little did I know that 25 years later, this younger man I married was to become my trials and tribulations in a devastating journey. Everyone used to say, "Beecher will get older, but he will never grow up." And I used to say "Well, I've spent my life raising kids, but I'll spend the rest of my life raising Beecher." How little did I know that someday that saying would come back to haunt me.

As a married couple we had quite a social life. He was heavily involved in the Elks Lodge, (a fraternal organization), and we spent a lot of time there as he went through the chairs and finally became Exalted Ruler. We both had good jobs and we did a lot of personal growth seminars. He was very articulate, as he had to be to present countless speeches at conventions etc. He was very good at it and he was a favorite among many people who trusted in his ideas. He was known by many, especially my family, as "Beecher the Preacher." He was everyone's "Savior" and he relished in the idea when he helped people. He expected nothing in return; he was just glad to help. My daughter Michelle always said, "God broke the mold when he made Beecher." He was so influential in both of my daughters' lives. He became the family's hero.

We enjoyed our lives and did a lot of traveling whenever we got the chance. Until I met him, I had never been anywhere, except California, Oklahoma and Hawaii. The many fishing trips to Cabo, Costa Rica, Acapulco, British Columbia and Hawaii again, were to me a sign of being successful and also a lot of fun! During the early years together, we got involved in a personal growth company, and we seemed to evolve into inspirational speakers. We both wanted to help others grow and be successful. To do this, we became Certified Firewalk Instructors. Yes, we taught people to walk across hot coals barefoot! We had our own company, Trails of Fire, a Goal Setting Seminar and we changed many lives! Becoming a motivational speaker, opened up new worlds for me as I never thought of myself as a person that could get up in front a group and speak with inspiration, inflection, and passion. But I did, and for six years we held our classes each month as we both continued working our day jobs. Needless to say, we finally got burned out. (No pun intended!)

As the years flew by, I made a few changes in my career and we even moved to Arizona for a few years. Beecher had a very high IQ and could memorize and talk up a storm about anything, sometimes way over my head. I guess I have quite a normal IQ, and sometimes I felt a little insecure that I could not retain everything I read like he could. He had the gift of gab, I guess you could say. He was good at his work, having been in the asphalt business most of his adult life after his service in the Seabees. He was well respected by his customers and his employers. But he could also spend money like crazy and we fought a lot about the spending. I was the more rational one always wanting to put money away for the future. If he had it in his pocket, he wanted to spend it. He was never greedy or selfish; he just wanted to help people and spending seemed to be a way of making him feel good as he had such a hard childhood. Having a mother that had been married thirteen times, he had many step fathers and step mothers as you can guess.

Our marriage had some ups and downs like most marriages do and there were several times we talked about divorce. He had a temper but most was verbal or emotional. Many times, he threatened to leave or divorce me, but he never followed through. Whenever I turned the table on him and said I was leaving, he begged me to stay as he did not want to be abandoned.

Shortly before I met Beecher, I had been seeing a counselor to help me understand why I kept choosing the wrong type of mate. She advised me not to tell Beecher because it would make me sound weak and he needed to know my strengths instead. After several months of always being late getting home on Tuesdays (my meetings with her were from 6:00-7:00 pm), I finally told him. I guess he thought I was seeing someone else. LOL!

Eventually we moved in together. It seemed a perfect situation. My daughters adored him and my youngest daughter was glad to have a real step father. They got along great. Then all of a sudden, he asked for my counselor's name and said he would like to talk to her himself. A few situations occurred just before this. My tires got slashed in the back-parking lot in the apartment where we lived and the same night, I received a call from an unknown woman who suggested I was sleeping with her husband. To this day, I do not know who the woman was or how she got my number. I figured she might have found an old piece of paper with my number on it. Must have been someone from my past as I was not seeing anyone but Beecher.

Shortly after that, Thanksgiving came around and he decided to go home to West Virginia to visit his family. I was not invited. It broke my heart. When he came back, he was somewhat distant. Shortly after that, we broke up. He said his counselor told him he needed to spend some time alone since he had not really lived by himself for very long after his divorce. Eventually we got back together and he proposed and we married in June 1991. We were very happy and bought our first home together the following year. He loved working in the yard and he excelled in his career and I did in mine.

Around 1994, he started having some health issues. Over a period of about five years, he had four knee surgeries which ended with a knee replacement, two back surgeries, and a gallbladder removal and a hemorrhoidectomy. Throughout this time, he became addicted to pain pills. He had always had migraine headaches, so he was always taking some kind of pill for that. The surgeries didn't help the addiction. Eventually he went into recovery and got very involved with NA (Narcotics Anonymous). He was drug free for over eight years and then one day the nightmare of FTD struck him. It came on like a slow-moving storm and burst into a hurricane over the next few years. I remember the day well. The storm didn't really come into full force until 2013, but the years leading up to that day are summed up in the following paragraphs.

Backtrack to 2008. We had moved to Arizona for a few years because of his job transfer. Nine months after the move, he lost his job. For the next year, he dabbled in trying to make a business involving increasing gas mileage on cars. He went on unemployment and we survived by using all of his 401K until broke and losing our home. He finally got a job back in Vegas and he commuted every day for about three months. He started staying with my daughters for several days a week rather than driving back and forth each way each day. Eventually our house foreclosed and we moved back to Vegas into a rental. By this time, we had lost our home in Las Vegas and our home in Arizona. After eighteen years of being a homeowner, we were now living in a rental and didn't see any indication of purchasing a home again. His new job did not provide the kind of income we were used to. Since I was close to Social Security age, I had to start drawing my Social Security to survive. Before we moved to Arizona, he had me retire from my job as an aesthetician and I had not renewed my license. I would have had to go through the whole process again to get my license.

Just before we left Arizona, I found out I had breast cancer. I had surgery and went through radiation once we moved back to Las Vegas in November. It was 2010 and as the year flew by to 2011, I started noticing some changes in Beecher but I couldn't put my finger on what it was. Later in the year, Beecher started becoming somewhat anti-social and distant with me. Some of our friends and family even noticed it. I think we all thought it was the stress of losing his job and having to move back to Las Vegas and the failures he felt.

During 2011, Beecher's stepmom passed away. He went back to West Virginia for the funeral. He seemed okay but a little distant. We settled into our new life in our rented home, made some new friends, and I started watercolor classes at the Club. My daughter Michelle had moved to Oregon in 2010 but moved back. I started going to a lot of craft shows to sell my foot jewelry which was very profitable. I joined the Race for the Cure for breast cancer and Beecher walked with me and our friends, Paul & Debbie and my sister-in-law Christine.

In May, Beecher was inducted into the Helldorado Hall of Fame in the Rodeo Division for his outstanding contributions to the Helldorado

Days Festival. Helldorado Days is an annual festival in Las Vegas, Nevada that hosts a rodeo, parade and a carnival. It is an organized event by the Elks Lodge as a fund raiser for local charities. Beecher was presented with a beautiful plaque. He was so proud and I was so happy for him. He deserved it for all his years in the Elks Lodge and his time invested in Helldorado.

We spent our 20th Anniversary in Newport Beach, California. Our favorite getaway place! Also, visited his step daughter Kimmie and grandkids in San Diego. It was a great weekend! 2011 also included a trip to Arizona to visit his nephews and a trip to Utah to visit my granddaughter, Bekkah for her birthday. It was also the year my oldest brother, Gary, turned 70 and we drove to Elko, Nevada in August to celebrate with my youngest brother Ricky and his wife Chris. It was on this trip that I started noticing some unusual changes in him. I think Ricky noticed it too.

In September I flew to California for my annual trip to visit my sister Linda for a week which included a wine trip to Yountville and to Lake Tahoe! It was one of the most relaxing weeks I've had, but little did I know it would be the last one for quite a while. It was also the year that I turned 65 and got an unexpected visit from my oldest best friend, Susie and her husband from Texas. We also went to a Golf Getaway in Mesquite, NV where I bet Miss Nevada, Alana Lee. She fell in love with my foot jewelry and I was honored to custom design my foot jewelry for all her dresses on the upcoming Miss America Pageant in January 2012! Beecher also received his 25-year pin from the Elks Lodge! It was one of the most memorable years as far as trips, craft shows, celebrations, parties and a lot of music events that included my youngest daughter Amy launching her music career by forming her own tribute act to the Black-Eyed Peas called the Black-Eyed Tease. Also, Michelle and her husband Cole moved back to Vegas from Oregon. All in all, 2011 was a very good year! 2012 presented more unusual changes in Beecher.

CHAPTER 2
2012—THE YEAR OF THE DRAGON
BEGINNING OF THE MAYAN CALENDAR

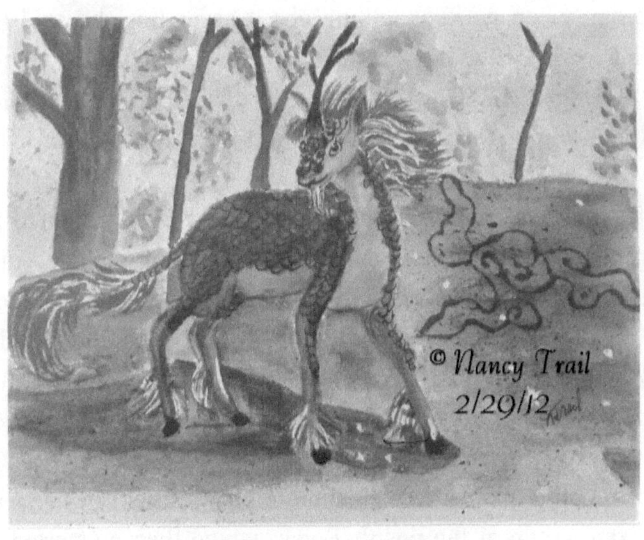

"The Year of the Dragon"
Watercolor by Nancy Trail
*"The dragon with his fire-breathing nostrils represents
aggressive connotations and corruption"*

The firestorm started brewing in 2012, when the Dragon reared its ugly head, but it would be over a year before the Snake slithered into our lives.

This was the year that almost did it for me as far as our marriage goes. In February he started attending some meditation meetings that were focused on the Mayan calendar. December 21st was supposed to be the end of the Mayan calendar and he started having some weird fascination about the world ending and or that he was going to ascend on that day. He tried to get me involved. I went to a few meetings but realized these people were in it for the money. They never charged but they always asked for donations. And these meetings started turning into being about people that had been abducted by aliens, healers or psychics. He now wanted to be a Healer and then he said he wanted to be a Psychic. I told him he couldn't just become Psychic; he had to be born one. One day when he kept talking about ascending, he said he would only have to work three days instead of five. I asked him where he was going to ascend to, and he put both of his hands up in the air and with a confused look on his face, he said, "I don't know." I told him if he didn't know he sure couldn't expect me to know.

The frustrations continued to mount as he started going to meetings every night that he didn't have NA meetings, which included our Friday night date night. This was seven nights a week he was at some kind of meeting. He didn't seem to care. He told me if I wanted to be with him, I could go to these meditation meetings with him. I started getting very frustrated with him and I felt he was being brainwashed by these people. I talked to his NA sponsor and he said to just keep on eye on him. He was still attending his NA classes three nights a week. In fact, he was in charge of one group at the hospital near us and then he started having a weekly meeting in our home. These were all fine. He had already been deeply involved with NA, and was helping other addicts and he needed these meetings to stay clean.

At this point in my story, you may wonder what all the definitions are about at the beginning of this story. Well, he was an "addict," addicted to pain pills. He sometimes said he believed he had been seeded here from another planet and was going to return to it. i.e., "alien." I, myself am considered a "normie" since I am not dependent on drugs or alcohol.

On September 24th, he got into another car accident for following too close. He told me he had stopped at a convenience store to get coconut water. He was trying to open it with a knife while driving and rear ended someone. Really? You've got to be kidding!

Sometime in October, he came home from his NA meeting and told me when he started to speak, the words would not come out. He knew them in his head, but they wouldn't come out of his mouth. Several weeks later, he mentioned the same thing. He said he thought it was bad demons at the hospital where he had his meeting. I laughed it off as I thought this was so called brainwashing. He said maybe he should see a doctor. We decided to wait until January. We had not paid any of our deductible for health insurance that year and would have to start over after New Year's. At this point in our marriage, I was ready to throw in the towel. I told him that after Dec. 21st, if the world didn't end, he was to stop all this nonsense. He agreed.

Dec. 21st rolled around and the world didn't end. But the next day he told me he had to go to a meeting. I asked him, "What for?" He said it was for the start of the new Mayan Calendar. I just about flipped out but decided what the heck? Christmas was in a few days, the family was coming over Christmas Eve, and I just wanted to get through the end of the year.

He came home from the meeting several hours later and had spent $60 money on an aura reading. Money was tight and I was furious! I told him I wanted a divorce, and I wanted him out of the house by January 1st. I told him he wasn't taking our dog Cammie either; she belonged to me. Also, he was not to have any communication with any of my family, including my daughters, one of whom he had raised. He did not seem bothered by any of this.

Within several hours, he had texted both of my daughters and very calmly told them we were getting divorced. Immediately, they called me and we decided to have an intervention with him. We decided on Christmas Eve since they were coming over anyway. For quite some time, they had noticed some changes in him. He had been very antisocial for quite some time, never hugging them hello and always playing games on his iPhone. They told me they had even talked amongst themselves about the fact that maybe he was having an affair. We had all been dumbfounded about his demeanor for quite some time. We had the intervention and we both compromised. He would cut down on his meetings to two a week and he would see his doctor in January. We all shed many tears, as we knew a storm was brewing. We just didn't know what was happening to him. We got through the holidays without any disruptions.

CHAPTER 3
2013—THE YEAR OF THE SNAKE
THE YEAR OF THE DIAGNOSIS

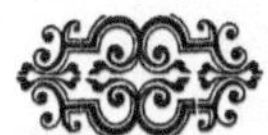

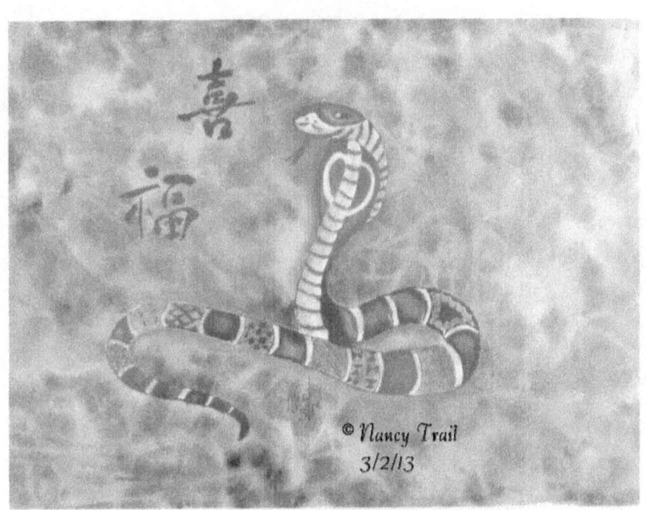

"The Year of the Snake"
Watercolor by Nancy Trail
"Snakes shed their skin and represent new beginnings but are also associated with negative and positive duality. They have a mysteriousness and indifference about them."

As the snake slithered into our lives and the unknown disease with it, we were met with confusion and unbelievable devastation to life as we knew it.

On January 2, Beecher called and made an appointment with his primary doctor. I met him there. We explained what had been going on. Beecher told the doctor about the problems in speaking. We all thought maybe he had had a stroke in his sleep. He referred him to a neurologist. Several weeks later, we visited the neurologist and he ordered an MRI and an EEG. Neither one showed any indication of a problem. By this time, about six weeks later, the neurologist referred him to a speech therapist. His speech was becoming worse, often leaving out words in a sentence.

For the next two months he saw a speech therapist twice a week as his speech continued to get worse. She sent him back to the neurologist and he said, there was no reason to continue to see him, as all the test results had proven inconclusive of any problems. Just before we left the doctor's office, Beecher pointed his finger at the doctor and somewhat stuttered the words, "You need to see a doctor because you have a bad heart."

The doctor looked at me in amazement and I just shook my head. I don't know where that came from, but as we left that day I was dumbfounded as I knew something was wrong with him and did not know where to turn for help. (And the doctor said there was nothing wrong with him?) I later learned that a lot of neurologists are not familiar with the type of disease that my husband was finally diagnosed with. It is specialized and rare.

Backtrack to January 7th. Beecher got a ticket for crossing over the double line on the express lanes on the freeway. In March he hit a curb near our house and ruined two tires on the left side of his car. Not enough to claim on insurance but still costing us almost $500 for two new tires. These tickets and accidents are starting to add up!

Also, sometime this month he kept telling me that all the lights were green driving to work all day. Later I would find a notebook where he had stated the same thing. And later he would often say it when we were driving somewhere after he lost his ability to drive. He seemed obsessed with the fact and he often laughed as if it were a game. I believe it to be part of his obsessions with his meditation groups and his ascension.

By the middle of April his speech was getting worse. He has had several minor car accidents and his driving is starting to scare me somewhat. I do most of the driving except he still continues to drive to work. He has to in order to keep his job which requires a lot of driving. I am now becoming scared of what is happening to him and me. I called and made an appointment with our old therapist that we had gone to see many years ago while he was having problems with addiction. She recommended that I make an appointment with the Cleveland Clinic Lou Ruvo Center for Brain Health here in Las Vegas (herein referred to as the Brain Center.) I called them and they told me to write a letter to them indicating the problems he was having and to please consider him for an evaluation. All I knew about the Brain Center at that time was it was for Alzheimer's and Parkinson's patients.

I wrote a letter telling them what had been going on and they set an appointment with Dr. Gabriel Léger. The earliest he could get into see him was May 30th. As I write this, I remember the time when we were living in Arizona, and we had come to Vegas to visit family. Beecher insisted we drive downtown to show me a building that had just been built and he thought was quite unusual. I had taken a picture of it and put it in my album that year and made the remark "Weird building." It was the Brain Center. Little did either of us ever envision that he would be a patient there some day.

Although his speech was slowly changing and he talked less, he still participated in certain events. In May, he walked with me in the Race for the Cure and we went to see Elton John at Caesars Palace. On May 12th (Mother's Day), he drove to the nearby store to get three items and on the way home he hit the curb and some bushes, resulting in damage of two tires again and scraping the whole left side of his car. This one we had to turn into the insurance. Glad no one else was involved. When I asked him how it happened, he said, "I was looking at the piece of paper you gave me with the three items you needed and wanted to make sure I didn't forget something." Three items and he couldn't remember! I was so angry at him. My daughters were on their way over to celebrate Mother's Day and I couldn't stop crying.

Another thing that was annoying me was the use of his debit card and his obsession with PCH (Publisher's Clearing House.) He played daily and didn't pay attention to what he was doing and often ordered items that were not needed. I soon found out what he was doing and I called PCH and told them the situation with my husband. They put a block on his account and closed it so he could not order any more items. They put "opted out" due to dementia. They removed him from the general mailing list. PCH was very nice and told me to keep the items (they weren't worth that much.)

My husband was 6'2" and at this time he now weighed 257 lbs. He started gorging his food and he ate ice cream like it was going out of style. He was way over his normal weight which was around 220 at the most. The only meds he was taking at this time were Amlodipine 5Mg. for high blood pressure and Trazodone (50Mg) for sleeping.

May 30 was his first appointment at the Brain Center. Beecher's doctor is Dr. Léger, one of a very few fellowship-trained behavioral neurologists in Las Vegas. Dr. Léger determined from some of the tests that he definitely had some difficulties with expression and understanding, progressive difficulties with language and also mild changes in personality, but overall good cognitive function. By this time, I had noticed more changes in his speech; shorter sentences, fewer words to describe things, preferring to use nouns and verbs and avoiding conjunctions. As he was in sales for an asphalt company, he was not "getting in the numbers" and his boss had requested a meeting with him about this. There was also mild stuttering and a tendency to rush answers with a" yes" when he meant "no" and "no" when he meant "yes." Sometimes I would jokingly say "Why don't you just say maybe." He also had difficulties naming certain objects such as naming a "squeegee" (a tool used in the asphalt business) which he now referred to as a "basting brush."

There were also behavioral changes and he tended to avoid social interactions, in part because of his difficulties speaking. In addition to the speech problem, he had always enjoyed cooking but he cooked less and had developed some ritualistic behaviors such as cleaning the table and stacking the dishwasher in an almost driven fashion, often before I had finished eating. I remembered thinking. "Gee it only took me 22 years to get him trained!" He also started doing his laundry every two or three days, which I had always done once a week on Sunday. His eating habits had changed a lot, tending to eat mostly sweets, especially ice cream which is why he had gained so much weight. He always gorged his food so fast he sometimes choked on it. He also seemed to urinate more frequently, sometimes ten times or more within a few minutes if we were out for the evening.

The best diagnosis Dr. Léger could give us at this time was "primary progressive aphasia" (PPA) which is loss of speech. A stroke was ruled out at this time. With a stroke, a patient's speech generally stays the same or gets better, but in Beecher's case it had continued to get worse. I wish it had been a stroke. We could have handled that better. The problem with PPA is that the patient has difficulties expressing himself and he starts withdrawing from life. He can quit talking altogether, avoid phone calls to friends and in turn friends quit calling because they don't know what to say to the patient. It alienates and creates a distance and eventually one loses his or her identity. Dr. Léger said it is often caused by some other process like Frontotemporal Degeneration (FTD or Pick's disease) but it was too early to tell. Primary Progressive Aphasia gradually robs people of their language skills while keeping their minds intact and it is degenerative. Unlike other degenerative conditions, like Alzheimer's, it leaves most of the patient's mental faculties untouched. Their memories stay healthy and their personalities remain unchanged, at least at first. Most aphasias are caused by trauma or stroke, which can improve over time but with PPA it never gets better. The inability to write, read, speak and comprehend can leave a patient locked inside his own head. I had noticed for quite some time, that Beecher was no longer the avid reader that he used to be. He had been a speed reader and could generally read a book in two sittings and retaining everything including Quantum Physics. Now he barely picked a book up.

To complicate matters, there are three types of variants of PPA, agrammatic, logopenic and semantic. His was agrammatic, which is a problem producing the words. He can remember the words but he struggles to speak them and string sentences together. Also, there is no cure for PPA and speech therapy is often recommended but Beecher had already been there and done that and there was no improvement. Later in the disease, he would often stutter and eventually his voice became soft and almost to a whisper. Many PPA patients often turn to hobbies that don't involve language which in Beecher's case later turned out to be painting with watercolors. Dr. Léger suggested he undergo neuropsychological testing and set up an appointment at the Brain Center for September 13, the earliest they could get him in. Three and a half months away! As I witnessed my husband slowly slipping away from me, I didn't know how much more I could take. I wanted answers and a cure. Little did I know what was to come.

I went home and spent hours and hours looking up this strange disease FTD and Pick's disease (another name for FTD), that I had never heard of. As time went on, I found out that nobody I knew had ever heard of it either. The best way to describe FTD is to say that the frontal lobe is shriveling up because brain cells are dying off. FTD is a form of behavioral variant that is marked by a loss of empathy and judgment. Later I would learn that Beecher had bvFTD which is the behavioral variant type. I was devastated when I found out the medical field did not know what caused it and there was no cure! As of now, it is estimated that at least 50,000-60,000 Americans currently suffer from some form of FTD. It is also the most common form of dementia in people under the age of 60, affecting the frontal and temporal parts of the brain, that are associated with organizational ability, decision making, judgment, self-control, emotional responsiveness, and language and comprehension. Some of them develop movement disorders that resemble Parkinson's disease. They may lack judgment and lose their ability for empathy, as well as have strong cravings for sweets. I hoped and prayed that this wasn't the case, but we would not know anything more for over three months.

Looking back, I remember when I had breast cancer in 2010, he didn't seem to be very worried or attentive to me and knowing what I now know, I think this disease started many more years ago than what we originally thought. Also, there were so many variations of the disease (no two people alike). The next morning, after the visit with Dr. Léger, Beecher said, I don't like the word "progressive" and we both knew it only got worse and not better. That was a culture shock to both of us. June 10, he got another ticket for running a red light on a left- hand turn. June 12, he got into another accident as he was pulling out of a parking lot near the same entrance to the freeway as before. Thank goodness no one got hurt.

On June 15th, we celebrated our 22nd wedding anniversary in the mountains for the weekend at our favorite hotel. We did some hiking and he seemed to enjoy that. During the hike, he stopped at a tree and carved our initials and the date in it. I realized at this time how distant he was becoming. Carving our initials and date in that tree gave me some hope but intimacy was starting to become a thing of the past.

We had started attending a church near our home. He loved it because they had a band and he really got into the music. June 30, he was baptized. It was something he wanted to do and I was so happy for him. Shortly after that we quit going to the church because he was starting to make people uncomfortable. He was approaching women he didn't know and was showing them pictures of our youngest daughter who is an entertainer. To this day, I don't know if maybe he had said anything sexual to them.

During the next few months, he had a few more small accidents in his car. Once when he was driving a few of his friends to a NA meeting, someone swiped him on the right side of his car and then took off. So, he said. They took a picture of the license plate but it didn't show up clearly. And then again on another day (I don't even remember the date), he ran into one of those cement blocks at a convenience store. It put a dent in the back of his car. I told him he was going to have to live with that as long as it still opened and closed. His boss expressed concern on his performance and took us to lunch to tell us he wasn't sure how long he could keep Beecher on. We begged him to keep him at least until he saw the doctor again in September. He agreed to do so as he liked Beecher and they were not only employee/employer but friends as well.

On July 2, he had a CT and PET scan ordered by Dr. Léger. They showed a minimal volume loss within the anterior left temporal lobe compared to the right. The findings suggested the possibility of semantic dementia, a form of frontotemporal dementia.

July 4th weekend we spent with some very close friends, Jim and Kathy at their cabin in Mammoth Lake, Utah. Four wonderful days relaxing! Beecher went trout fishing every day, and I got to enjoy time relaxing by the stream that ran through the back of their property. I got to do some plein air (outdoor) painting for the first time. Beecher was just happy to be fishing and eating trout tacos! Other than not talking much, he was often clumsy and I had to keep an eye on him. I hated to go home and back to the life we now had. But I was so thankful for the trip as it was one of the happiest times, we had that year.

On July 16 (my oldest brother's birthday), Beecher had an accident on the way home from work. He went to the hospital because he complained of his neck hurting. While lying on the gurney, he told me he could no longer drive and I agreed with him. His car was totaled and he had hurt another person. He did not seem to care that he could no longer drive. He was released from the hospital with only a little whiplash. (The next two years turned into a nightmare for me as the lady he hit decided to sue us). She had minor injuries but she took it to the limit on our insurance policy. I had been with our insurance company for over 28 years but they cancelled our policy because of all of Beecher's accidents and tickets. However, they had to pay for the accident. So of course, I had to find another insurance company and of course it was higher but at least we only had my car to insure. That's another story for another time but not in this book.

As of this date, Beecher has had eight car accidents and three moving violations since November of 2011, which is about an 18-month time frame! It's a miracle he didn't kill himself or someone else or me for that matter. With all the tickets, accidents, ticket doctors, deductibles since November 2011, it cost us in excess of $5000! Without a car and unable to drive, his boss let him continue to work mostly in the office and some of the other salesmen would take him out in the field. I would drive and pick him up and on Saturdays I would drive him out to measure parking lots. I knew his time was running short but I hung on hoping that his upcoming appointment in September would give us a better answer as to his diagnosis. I was just dreaming. I didn't know how we would survive without his paycheck. We had no savings. He had spent all of his 401K in Arizona and the only income I had was my Social Security I had started receiving in 2011. I envisioned us moving in with my daughters.

On July 30, his boss called me and said he was going to have to let Beecher go. I asked him to please let him finish out the week and he agreed to wait until Monday, August 2, my oldest daughter's birthday. Why do all the bad things happen on my family's birthdays? I drove to his work and Beecher and I sat at his desk while his boss terminated his employment. Unemployment would now be our only other income. That turned out to be another battle for me, as his boss's wife turned in a false report and the unemployment office first denied it. She didn't much care for Beecher and she was heartless. It took several months to get it resolved. What saved us was the fact that she was not in the room at the time of the termination, but I was. It was just another battle in this ongoing saga.

The next few weeks were a blur as I tried to figure out how to survive before the unemployment kicked in. At $407 a week for 26 weeks, it did not compare to what he had been making. It seemed all I did was manage Cobra Insurance that replaced his insurance at work and was considerably more, unemployment, attorneys, and forms to fill out. We had to start paying the higher Cobra insurance in August. Sometime in September, I filed a claim for Beecher's Short -Term Disability. Initially it was denied and I had to contest it. Psychological conditions are not covered by our policy, except for Alzheimer's disease and other organic senile dementias. The claim was finally accepted and we were paid on it in April 2014. My oldest daughter Michelle set up a "Go Fund Me" account and we were lucky to have some great friends that came to our financial rescue.

The one stress reliever that I had was my watercolor class. I had been taking classes at our club house for several years. It was my escape and I looked forward to going every week for three hours. In August, since Beecher was no longer working, I started taking him to class with me. He started painting and really enjoyed it. He had quite a knack for it. He could paint twice as fast as me and was really doing well. The disease had affected his frontal temporal lobe which is language, organization and behavior. The other part of his brain that was not affected was the creative part; art, and music. The creative part seemed to take over in place of his language problems. His mentality was like a child; he didn't care about the end result. He just painted what he saw. Painting became something we did together and he relaxed and enjoyed showing off his paintings. He showed pride in what he painted.

September 23–Today was to become the beginning of the end of our normal life as we had known for 25 years. Never would our life be the same. The results were in after several hours of neuropsychological evaluation testing:

- Masked face, with decreased blinking
- Cognitive dysfunction
- Some degree of memory loss
- Behavioral changes including obsessive behaviors
- Became fixated on paranormal beliefs – perhaps an exaggeration of his earlier beliefs.
- He has had eight car accidents and surrendered his license.
- Language symptoms have worsened.
- Impairment of activities of daily living
- Disinhibition
- Changes in appetite and eating
- Very unlikely he will be able to return to work in any manner.

Dr. Léger stated that Beecher has a degenerative syndrome resulting in impairment of judgment, language and other cognitive functions.

Diagnosis – Because of the additional behavioral changes and the language impairments, this seems to most likely be consistent with a form of frontotemporal lobar degeneration (FTD) sometimes called Pick's disease and PPA – Primary Progressive Aphasia.

These are the words I dreaded. No hope for a cure and no indication of how long before this dreadful disease will take his life. No treatment planning of any kind. No idea what other symptoms will appear throughout the course of this disease. It's more wait and see and deal with it as it appears. With the Aphasia, most patients become mute at some point. The storm is brewing and I cannot see an end in sight. The doctor added a new medication – Quetiapine (Seroquel) to take at bedtime to help with sleep in addition to the Trazodone he is already taking.

I was referred to a social worker at the center under the Caregiver Counseling Program and also a support group. In addition to the Association for Frontotemporal Dementias (AFTD), I was also referred to the Cleveland Clinic in Ohio to request financial aid. And I was given a list of Advance Directives, i.e. Living Will, Durable Power of Attorney for Health Care, and Durable Power of Attorney for Finances, and a DNR (Do not Resuscitate Form) and information of an Elder Law Attorney. I felt like I was in a haze of a nightmare. How could this be happening?

Trying not to cry or let Beecher see me crying, I drove home in absolute devastation. I was already expecting the diagnosis but I did not want to believe it was happening to us. It was a death sentence in the worse way. My husband and best friend is slowly slipping away from me and there was nothing in the world I could do about it and I had no idea when he would be gone from me and this world. I had no idea of the toll it was going to take on me and my family. My dearly beloved husband was only 59!

Shortly after he was diagnosed, he wrote this in his own words on the computer:

October 18, 2013
"I hate Picks Disease"

I hate picks disease; it is causing me a lot of problems. Problems with my speck, problems with my life. I wrecked my car 5 times since I had picks disease. I finally totaled my car. I got laid off from my job for medical reasons. Totaled my car, life has thrown me for a loop.

Beecher

Soon after the shock starting wearing off, realizing our life would never be the same, I made an appointment to talk with the therapist in the Caregiver Counseling Program at the Brain Center. I knew I could not do this alone. The emotional stress was already getting to me, and especially the financial burden and already the feeling of grief and loss. My husband had already changed so much. I didn't understand my feelings or how to deal with situations that I felt were beyond my control. I spent most of my sessions with Jenna my counselor, crying my eyes out. After about four months, I actually made it through a session without crying.

I also started attending a Support Group which was led by Lisa Radin who with her son had written the book, "What if it's not Alzheimer's." Her husband had passed away from FTD fifteen years earlier. I was so glad to have her as my mentor and confidante and I looked forward to sharing my dilemma and story with others in the same sinking boat as me. We met once a month. Everyone's story was different but had the same end result and as we learned to try to cope with our situation, we all helped each other. I remember one gentleman, Howard, who had lost his wife seven months before, who still came to the meetings as he was still grieving. His input helped me face this devil of a nightmare. We all had questions like "What is the next stage and how long does it last?" No one had an answer since nobody knows and everyone is different. And "Did your loved one ever do this?" I remembered Howard telling me "Every six months, you will wish it was the six months before." I wasn't quite sure what that meant, but I figured it out. It seemed at least to me that things seemed to progress to a different level about every six months. Just when you thought some things had slowed down and adjusted to some of them, then all of a sudden, a bunch of new symptoms and situations appeared and it was time to adjust to them. I realized it had been easier the six months before. And yet, there was no going back. Thank God for Lisa to help me and guide me through this difficult time. It was not easy. The stress was unbearable! I started reading everything I could find on the subject and often attended the Lunch and Learn Program they had at the Brain Center.

My role as a caregiver was not what I had bargained for. It is very hard to retain your independence as your life and responsibilities have been affected, physically, emotionally and economically. While I tried to maintain the quality of life for my husband, I was busy keeping track of appointments with the doctors, medications and exercise. In the meantime, I also tried to show the love and support necessary to meet the many demands of this devastating disease. Every responsibility that you and your loved one used to share now becomes your full responsibility. Questions I asked myself were, "When do I start discussing my husband's wishes regarding a will and a DNR?" As we had already had a will in place and I knew he did not want to be resuscitated, it was still hard to bring up the subject, so I avoided it. I remember casually asking the doctor at one of his appointments, "What's the average time he will live?" The doctor casually remarked "Hopefully about eight years." I wasn't sure if my husband was really listening or understood what I had asked the doctor. Later that night after dinner, my husband said, "So the doctor said "I'm going to die in eight years?" I didn't know how to react so I just said, "No, he meant the average is eight years but you could live up to fifteen years or more." He seemed okay with that.

I also remember one time he started crying and said "I don't know what's wrong with me." Another time when I was crying and upset about something, he said, "I don't like it when you cry; it makes me sad and I don't know how to help." That brought me to my knees. I tried not to let him ever see me cry again. After that, I let out my emotions in the shower or when I chose to take a walk. Many times, my walks were taken to get out of the house and away from him for a few minutes while I calmed down about something he had done for the tenth time that day. One time he broke my favorite dish my mother had given me. I was so upset. It had shattered to pieces. Beecher was barefoot and I tried to get him to move out of the way to avoid him getting his feet cut, while I also swept up the pieces. When I finally accomplished that, I told him I was going to take a walk and he said, "I'll go with you." I shouted, "No, you're not!"

After my walk, I had cooled down. I sat down to talk to him. He said "I don't like it when you yell at me." I apologized and told him I wasn't mad at him. I was mad at the disease. I realized then that it wasn't his fault and I learned to handle my outbursts of emotions, or at least while in front of him. He was becoming so childlike and my role as a wife had started changing to the role of a mother. I did not like this new role and kept wondering, "Where did my husband go?'

The subject of sex was a difficult one. It was becoming mundane for me. It was always to please him and I got no satisfaction as I felt like I was having sex with a stranger. It was a very uncomfortable feeling. I talked with my counselor about it and finally made a decision to talk to Beecher about it. Finally, after sex one night, I knew I had met my limit to time in the bedroom. The next morning, I told him I no longer wanted to make love to him. It just about broke my heart to tell him. I told him it was very uncomfortable for me because I always got a UTI after and it sometimes took days to clear up. (Sometimes, you have to lie a little but it was true on many occasions.) I told him I had to be in the best health so I could continue to take care of him and if I am having an episode with a urinary tract infection, I didn't feel good enough to take care of him. He seemed to accept it and that was the last time we made love –if you want to call it that. That little conversation took a load off of me and I was glad I had made that decision. To be fully truthful, Beecher had developed Herpes many years before we met, but he was always cautious and would let me know if he felt an episode coming on and we would avoid sex until it passed. With his disease, I also feared he would not be so respectful or cautious, and that scared me as well, so I felt in my heart it was a good decision. Whew, glad to get that off my chest!

2013 was filled with a lot of visits from friends and family. Beecher's sister came to visit in February from Ohio and my brother from Northern California. My granddaughters came from Utah in June and my sister Linda in August also visited. In October our good friend Bret from Seattle was in town for the weekend and we spent time out eating, gambling and a trip to Sam's Club where he bought us a new TV since ours had gone out. My good friend Sue from California also came and helped me out with one of my craft shows. In between waiting for doctor appointments and diagnosis, I managed to attend quite a few craft shows where I sold my foot jewelry which also brought in some much-needed money.

November was not a good month, although there has not been a good month since this nightmare started. I rear ended someone while delivering an item I had sold on Craigslist. Instead of waiting for them to pick it up the next day I agreed to deliver it to them. I was desperate to get anything sold. I hadn't had a ticket or accident in over 20 years. Guess this is what stress does to you. It was also the month that our dearly beloved Shih Tzu, Cammie died on the day after Thanksgiving. We were blessed to have had her for 12 ½ years and we were devastated. We ended off the year in December with a plane ride to Seligman AZ for breakfast with our good friends, Jimmy and Kathy who owned their own small plane. Beecher was excited because he got to fly and land the plane with the help of Jimmy. Scary! First time in a small plane but it was a lot of fun!

We paid the last Cobra payment and starting in January we would be on Obama Care. At least it will be cheaper than Cobra.

The highlight of 2013 was our biggest and most entertaining experiences in one year. My youngest daughter Amy had started performing in her own band called Black Eyed Tease and we went to several of her performances. Her boyfriend belonged to a band called Raiding the Rock Vault. We attended that show seven times that year. Of course, we always got free tickets!

As money was tight, I was doing everything I could to bring in extra cash. I had started going through all the items in our house and garage that I could sell to make money. Little did I know that eBay and Craigslist were going to become my best friends in the next year or so. Going back to work was unthinkable as I was finding it difficult to leave Beecher alone for any length of time. Plus taking him with me was often hard.

Friends suggested I look into an Adult Day Care. One day after his doctor appointment, I took him to look into one near our home. I was so sure he wouldn't want to go but what did I have to lose? To prepare him, I told him there was a place he could go where they had activities like bingo and singing. We walked in and to my amazement he seemed interested! At least he didn't turn around and walk out. I showed him the library where he could sit and read or play his games with his iPad. Several activities were going on and he looked around. Next was the kitchen. The cooks were preparing lunch. He walked over and helped himself to a bread roll and then a doughnut left from breakfast. This was a good sign since he loved to eat, especially carbs and donuts. We went in to talk to the director about what I needed to do for admission. I asked him if he wanted to come there one day a week and he nodded and said yes. I had no idea it would be so easy. I was so relieved as I thought I would have to battle with him to make this work. The fact that most of the people were well into their 70's or older didn't seem to bother him.

In January I would get this process started. Since he was a veteran, I had already applied for VA Disability Compensation under non-service-connected veterans which made him eligible for VA Health Benefit. They placed him in Priority Group #5 that included the Basic Medical Benefits Package, Mental Health, Home Health Care, Geriatrics and Extended Care, Nursing Home Placement, & Mileage Reimbursement. Under Geriatrics, the Respite Care Program which was for the Caregivers, there was included a 5 day stay in an approved Facility and Adult Day Care for him. The respite care services are available up to 30 days per year on a minimum five-day respite care in a facility for the patient which gives the caregiver time to relax from the normal grind of taking care of a loved one on a 24/7 basis. Respite is a fancy word for "giving you a break." I was soon to learn I would need many days of respite. I would encourage every caregiver to seek respite care. Feelings of resentment are normal and I found myself frustrated and sometimes hating him. I didn't realize this early in the diagnosis that I resented him for being sick; I felt sorry for both of us. It was eerie sometimes when I looked at him with his masked face. He never seemed to blink and people often thought he looked weird. The blank stare often frightened people and they didn't want to be around him.

As I look back at this past year, I remember Dr. Léger asking me when I first noticed a subtle change in Beecher. I told him when Beecher started becoming antisocial somewhere around 2011 or 2012. The one thing that I had not recalled until recently was a night in June 2012 when we had gone to a concert to see a friend of ours, Michael Grimm perform at Sunset Station. In addition, another friend of ours, Curt was playing in the band. My daughter Amy and her friend Stephanie met us there. We were enjoying the show and dancing quite a bit. Beecher didn't usually dance much to slow music, but that night, he couldn't seem to get enough. A long time ago, I had casually mentioned to him, that he never looked at me when we were dancing. But that night he had a Cheshire grin on his face the entire night and he constantly stepped on my toes. He wanted to dance every dance, fast or slow. I remember the strange look in his eyes and the grin on his face almost scared me. I got to the point that I quit dancing with him, because my feet were getting stomped on so much! Looking back at that night, I realized there were more changes than I had originally thought. I now realize something was going on with him back then.

Another thing that I recalled was in August this year. I bought a birthday card for my oldest half-brother, Gary. I asked Beecher if he wanted to write something in his card. For some reason I had taken a picture of the card when I put it in my 2013 album and just recently saw it as I was looking through the album. This is what he wrote:

Beech

Gary, I love you. I like port wine. You're a good friend.

What is so unusual about this is that he signed his name first instead of after. The mention of the port wine was from a visit we had taken to visit my brother, Gary on his 70th birthday in Elko in 2011. We had driven to Elko for the weekend to celebrate. Beecher was never a drinker, but he got turned on to port wine, and he drank a lot with my brother. After we got home from the trip, he kept buying port wine for quite a while. Also, the fact that he said, "You're a good friend" instead of a good brother. It's weird not being able to piece things together, but that's the sadness of FTD. Things were already getting mixed up in his brain besides losing his speech. Beecher had not been diagnosed at this time in August. He wasn't diagnosed until September.

The year ended off with Christmas Eve at our house with family and our good friends, Dave and Anita. All in all, we had made some wonderful memories in spite of the disease and we realized how grateful we were to have such amazing friends and family.

CHAPTER 4

2014—THE YEAR OF THE HORSE
JOURNALING TO DEAL WITH MY FRUSTRATIONS

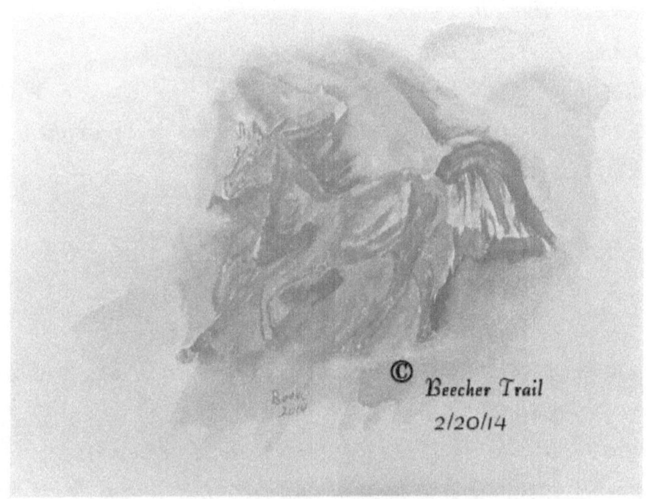

"The Year of the Horse"
Watercolor by Beecher Trail
"Horses represent intellectual spirit, drive, passion and an appetite for freedom and give you a strong motivation that carries one through life"

As I started writing in a journal this year, I realized how it helped deal with my frustrations. I downloaded an app called "Werd-smith" on my iPhone and it was easy to journal every day or evening or wherever I was at the time. Later, I would just send it to my computer and forward it to Microsoft Word. While Beecher continued to decline, I wrote down my feelings. It felt good to vent since I didn't want to keep yelling at him all the time. Here are some of the habits he started developing:

Habits:

Picks teeth constantly with those little blue toothpicks that I nicknamed little Blue Gremlins as they appeared everywhere and he always had one in his mouth

Does everything in a hurry

Doesn't finish tasks that he starts

Spills things all the time

Doesn't finish completely washing silverware and puts them in the drawer still dirty

Nighttime Habits:

- *Combs hair before going to bed*
- *Instead of wearing t-shirts daily, he puts on dress shirts as if he's going to work*
- *Household chores: dishes, laundry; he is very messy*
- *Brushes his teeth and uses mouthwash five to ten times per day or more and usually misses the sink when he spits and he's not even aware of it.*
- *Yard work: blows all the leaves from our backyard into our neighbor's yard.*

January–started the process getting him into the Adult Day Care. The one we visited a few months ago was about fifteen minutes from our home and they would pick him up and bring him home. Included meals and activities and he would be gone for eight hours. Only problem was the cost, so I checked into applying for some grants. Since he had been diagnosed with FTD, I qualified for a grant from the AFTD organization as well as Alzheimer's and Helping Hands. I had to apply for each one separately which I did, and each grant could run consecutively after the first one. It took some time. He had to have a TB test. I had to set up his ride through RTC, our local Rapid Transit Co. (get his picture taken, get his card which he had to carry, call and set up an appointment time for the day before each pickup).

Since he had already been diagnosed with FTD, I contacted AFTD.org and started the application process. In the next few months, I would find out about the VA benefits.

AFTD grants were for $500 and since the cost of the ADC was $65 a day, that gave me seven days. I spread it over seven weeks which gave me one day a week. They approved me in a timely manner. Over the course of the next year and a half, I applied simultaneously with each organization to run back-to-back so that I didn't miss a week. The Alzheimer Organization had a $500 grant as well, but Helping Hands had $1000, which gave me fifteen days or three and a half months. The first grant started in March. I was thrilled to have a day to myself. When he left on the bus that first day, I sat in my favorite chair for several hours just enjoying the peace and quiet. I wasn't quite sure what to do; go shopping, get a pedicure, read to my heart's content without an interruption or just stay home and do nothing. I chose to do NOTHING! I almost felt guilty but not for very long.

Through the coming weeks, I started getting out of the house; going to the movies or lunch with my sister or friends. It felt great to be free of the burden of taking care of him 24/7. But I always made sure I was home at least an hour before he got home so I could just relax and have some peace and quiet. Some days I actually started getting what I thought might be a panic attack (I don't know because I've never had one, but I'm sure it was close to it). I didn't know whether to do things that needed to be done around the house so I wouldn't get interrupted once he got home or just sit and enjoy the quiet. It was usually the latter.

One day a week was more than I had before, but I soon found out it was not enough.

I soon found out from the VA that they would pay for Visiting Angels to come into my home for assistance. There were more forms to fill out but I soon got that approved after a home visit. They said they would pay for four hours, four days a week. I wasn't sure I would like strangers in my home, but they assured me they were all bonded. I could try it out and if I liked it, I could specify a certain one if I liked one better than the other. The first one I had for a couple of days. Okay, but not very friendly. The second one was definitely not to my liking. I was leery about leaving someone alone in my house, but I decided to try to get used to it, so I gave her instruction on what to do while I was gone. I went grocery shopping and was gone for less than an hour. I came back into the house through my garage. I guess she didn't hear me as I found her napping in my favorite chair. Strike two!

The next one I struck Gold with. She was the angel I had been hoping to find. Even though at this point I was still leery, she came back the second day and by the third day I was sure I wanted her. Not only that, she wanted us! She lived close by and she preferred to have one client as well, so I immediately told her boss and requested her on a permanent basis. She was willing to work at the times I needed her. I got to pick the days and hours I wanted her. I was in heaven and felt my prayers had been answered! She was not only the best caregiver, but she cooked, cleaned, played scrabble with my husband, and got him to read out loud to her on occasion. I could leave my house without worrying about her or him or I could just go escape into my office and make my phone calls and make jewelry without any interruption. Sometimes she even made soup at her home and brought it to us. In addition to that, she had been an EMT at one time and drove an ambulance so I was confident that she could handle any emergency. She eventually became one of my best friends, and I loved how dearly she took care of my husband. Her patience was unimaginable. I couldn't believe how lucky I was to have found her. I was now feeling confident that I could get through this dilemma now that I had Adult Day Care one day a week and had Frances (Beecher called her Franny the Nanny), four days a week for four hours. I felt that I could do this now!

~

January 15

First journal entry. This was a very upsetting day! After I got up and fixed breakfast for us, I went into my office to work on paying bills. Beecher walked into my office and very nonchalantly told me he tried to hang himself last night. I almost lost it! "What do you mean?" I asked him. He headed to the garage and showed me a satin karate belt that was still hanging over the garage shelf where it looked like he had attempted to do so. I could tell the rack wasn't high enough to accomplish the task. I asked him why but he did not respond. He just started taking the belt down. After we got back inside, I sat him down and asked him again. He finally said it was because I wouldn't get him another dog. I explained to him again the reason why. I told him I would not have liked to find him like that and he said he wouldn't do it again. I called and talked to his doctor and he said he would have the psychiatrist talk to him at his next visit in a few weeks. I was so upset I couldn't sleep that night, not knowing what he might do next.

Beecher has always owned several guns which he kept in the house in addition to a collection of knives. I immediately gathered them all up and hid them until I could find someone to buy them. Better to be safe than sorry. I would feel better once we got rid of the guns and knives. I hoped he would never attempt to do something this crazy again. What if he lost his temper and tried to hurt me? This disease was so crazy, I didn't know what to expect. Times of frustrations came and went like the hours on a clock, as we tried to understand this disease and what was happening to him.

After our dog Cammie died at the end of November, he constantly asked me about getting another dog. Every time we drove by the Animal Hospital where we took her after she passed away, he always said, "They killed my dog." I told him I couldn't get another dog because we couldn't afford it and it would be hard for me to take care of him and another dog.

~

January 20

Our watercolor teacher, Sylvia got our class into an Art Show at the Gallery at the Multigenerational Center for a one night showing. This was the first art show for Beecher. He was very excited about it. He entered a picture of a cat that he had painted. My daughter Amy and friends, Jim and Kathy, Dave and Anita, Paul and Debbie came to the showing. Beecher loved showing off his work. Fun night!

Beecher called a few of his friends regarding his guns. Beecher owed one of his friends about $6,000 from a $10,000 loan. He had borrowed the money several years ago when he was unemployed and he was trying to make a business work in Arizona. Beecher had never even told me he had borrowed the money until we had to start making payments to him. We had been making payments for about two years. His friend agreed to take one of the guns towards the debt. We will probably never be able to pay off the remaining balance but at least the gun went towards what we owed him. Two of his friends agreed to buy the others. We set up a time in the next few days to do the exchange. Will be glad to get that settled. Less to worry about. Will probably sell the knives on eBay.

~

February 24

Today I took Beecher to see Dr. Léger at the Brain Center. He also saw the Psychiatrist, Dr. Wint. Dr. Wint is also the NV Energy Chair for Brain Health Education. I had called Dr. Léger last week regarding Beecher's attempted suicide. Dr. Wint and Dr. Léger agreed his suicide attempt was more of a threat, but there is still impulsivity. Beecher denies suicidality at this time. Since his last visit, Dr. Léger felt Beecher's symptoms had worsened. Cognitive functions were much worse and there were changes in his voice. New meds were added. Tamsulosin (Flomax) to improve urination and Venlafaxine / Effexor an antidepressant. On Dr. Léger's office visit notes, he mentioned that the FTD was now considered bvFTD which is behavioral variant frontotemporal dementia.

March 4

I took Beecher to another visit to see Dr. Léger and Dr. Wint. When Dr. Wint asked him about the suicide attempt he said, "I tried to kill myself.' When asked why, he said, "I did it for attention. My wife is not sleeping with me anymore." When questioned further about the issue of a new dog, he said, "I want a dog. It's important to me." He doesn't seem to understand the financial burden and the caregiving it requires especially when I have so much to do taking care of him. After repeated reinforcement from Dr. Wint, he finally responded with, "I'm not going to get a dog. I just have to get used to it." They made some changes in his meds to reduce some of his problems. Dr. Wint is a very sincere doctor as well is Dr. Léger. As we were leaving, Dr.Wint said to me, "I don't know how most people deal with this disease. I commend you for being such a good caregiver. It must be devastating. It's like taking care of a 6'2" five-year-old." I agreed as I had thought that myself many times. That remark from Dr. Wint was very endearing to me.

March 7

Beecher's first day at Adult Day Care! Yay! The Alzheimer grant has been approved! Starting today Beecher will have seven weeks, and will go one day a week until April 18. Better than nothing!

March 15

St. Patrick's Day! Went to dinner and party at the Clubhouse. He was in a good mood and even danced a few dances with me without stepping on my feet!

~

March 20

I finished a quilt that I had been making for Beecher out of his old t-shirts. He was very happy that I had made it for him. I don't know how I had time to work on it. Guess I just needed something else to keep me busy.

~

March 22

We drove out to Pahrump to attend one of my best friend's Installation of Officers as Exalted Ruler of the Elks Lodge. She has been very involved for many years. It was a good day. Beecher did well but he was very quiet.

~

April 5

Started the day with a Craft Fair that started at 9 am until 2 pm. I had just found out a few days before that one of our favorite couples we knew when we lived in Bullhead City, Arizona had both died in a motorcycle accident. The funeral was the same day. I didn't want to miss it but I didn't want to cancel the fair as we needed the money. Franny helped me with that. Got up early, packed our clothes for the funeral as we were staying the night at a friend's house after the funeral, laid out clothes for Beecher, loaded my car for the craft fair. Then I called the lady at the fair who was in charge of the vendors and told her I needed to leave an hour early as it was an hour and a half drive to Laughlin where the funeral was. Normally if you leave an event early you are never invited back to participate again but under the circumstances, she approved it. Said my goodbye to Franny and off to the Craft Fair I went, then rushed home, unloaded my car, reloaded my car with suitcases. Franny had Beecher dressed and ready to a certain point. Said our goodbyes to Franny again and drove to Laughlin.

We got to Laughlin in enough time to ask one of my friend's husbands, to tie Beecher's tie. He had forgotten how to do it. Most of our friends had not seen Beecher since we moved but they knew of his illness and were very helpful and considerate. After the funeral, we went to our friend's house for the night. While there, Beecher somehow managed to break the toilet seat in the guest bathroom the morning we were leaving. I felt so bad but they told us not to worry about it. Before we drove back to Vegas, we visited Beecher's nephews who lived close by. They told me they noticed the changes in him and were very sad to see that.

~

April 13

My sister Linda came to visit from California. My other sister Patti took us to Lake Havasu which was about a two-and-half hour drive for a two-day sister getaway. My oldest daughter Michelle offered to come to the house to watch Beecher.

Everything seemed to be fine. Michelle said she had no problems with him except for cleaning up after him all the time, which seemed to be the norm but she handled it well.

The next day, she confessed to my younger daughter Amy that he had made a sexual offer to her. When she told him that wasn't nice, he then asked her if her friend would do the favor. He didn't say anything else and the subject was dropped. She did however lock the bedroom door that night just in case.

She was too embarrassed to tell me directly what he said. That is why she told Amy and then Amy told me. I talked to them both and explained that dis-inhibition was quite common in this disease. Since there was no intent to hurt, for them not to fear him. Just to let me know if it continued. There was never another incident.

The next day we took him to the Container Park and out to dinner at Hot N Juicy Crawfish. He liked both as usual.

While Linda was here, we took several long walks with him. Beecher usually walks ahead of me and always wants me to play the music from the group Bread with David Gates. He never asks for any other music.

Linda noticed that Beecher never looks when he crosses the streets. She told him, like she was telling a child, that he was supposed to look both ways before he crossed the street so he wouldn't get hit by cars. He was not even aware that he was doing it. We still had to remind him, as it went in one ear and out the other.

Today I found out after nine months, we finally got paid on the Short-Term Disability policy. The best news I've had in two years! Maybe we will survive financially after all.

∼

May 20

Visit with Dr. Léger. Beecher has lost a few pounds and blood pressure is good. Since last visit in March, Beecher's mood has been much better. He has been helpful with chores around the house and he has not been having any angry outbursts. I believe the new meds have helped.

He still has a strong desire for sweets and eats a lot of ice cream. He wolfs down his meal and sometimes does not finish before he starts looking for dessert. Doctor took him off the Effexor/ Venlafaxine and the Flomax. I guess he felt Beecher no longer needed them.

∼

May 23

Beecher had finally started receiving Social Security Disability Benefits in February this year. The AFTD grant kicked in and now Beecher has seven more weeks at Adult Day Care. Thank God! Another Alzheimer grant got approved and will kick in after that so now he can have Day Care until August 8.

Earlier in the year, I applied for VA benefits and at first was denied. Then I applied for a Hardship Determination which he finally got approved for. He was eligible for Health Benefits and it paid for everything except prescriptions. I found out at this time that the VA only approved one day per week for Adult Day Care. I was so disappointed that I could only get one day for him and the booklet from the VA did not indicate this. In an effort to push for more days in Adult Day Care, I wrote a letter to Harry Reid our Senator and several other politicians in Nevada and pleaded with them to do something about the VA program here in Las Vegas. The only response I got was that was the way it was in Nevada and that they would take the issue to Congress next time they were in session. The thing that upset me the most was that the Veterans Handbook said that he was entitled to Respite care on a daily basis. That never happened as I never got a response from them. They basically said Nevada doesn't have a program for five days like other states have and that the VA only pays for Vets on Pension but denies it to the rest. I explained that I knew that the VA pays a reduced fee to the Adult Day Care for some patients to attend and explained that I had done my homework and knew this to be a fact.

~

June 1–2

We had another art show at the Community Center where we lived. Beecher and I entered two paintings each. We both received a Certificate of Special Recognition for Participating in the Event. He was even more excited this time. He got a lot of compliments and one lady even offered to buy one of his paintings after the show was over. His face lit up! The next day we took it to her and she paid him for it. I told him he could keep the money and buy whatever he wanted. We went to the toy section of the store and he bought a checkers game and another small toy. So glad to see him so happy!

~

June 3-5

My 50th Reunion was held at three locations on three days here in Las Vegas. Graduation day was held at the football field of the new high school. This had not been done in many years as the graduation was usually held inside an auditorium. It was our high school's 100th year graduation and since we were celebrating 50 years we were invited to graduate with that class. Included were gold caps and gowns for all of us. It was an exciting time. Amy brought Beecher to it. No mishaps except constantly running him back and forth to the bathroom.

~

June 8

Our good friends, Jimmy, and Kathy, invited us to take a night flight in their small plane to a nearby Mesquite, NV casino for dinner. Fun night! Glad to be able to still share some wonderful memories with wonderful friends. As Beecher was losing much of his speech by now, he could still communicate when he needed to. They were very patient with him.

~

June 15

Our 23rd Anniversary and Father's Day were on the same day. We had all of the family over for dinner. Beecher did the usual, eat and play Angry

Birds on his iPad. Frances bought a card for me from Beecher and helped him sign it and he gave it to me along with a bottle of wine. Frances is so sweet and thoughtful.

June 20

I took Beecher to the movies to see "Jersey Boys." Great movie!

At the end he stood up and clapped his hands!

He really liked it and so did I.

The Brain Center set up a My Chart Caregiver website that I signed up for. It made it easier to communicate with the doctors and the nurses when I had questions that couldn't wait until the next appointment. They were always quite prompt in answering my questions.

July 1

Told Beecher I would make sausage and scrambled eggs for breakfast.

He asked me to put brown sugar on the eggs. I told him that wasn't a good idea. But he did it anyway.

Anything sweet, I guess.

July 4

I noticed some poop on the shower curtain in the guest bath. He doesn't know how it got there.

July 5

After dinner, he did dishes as usual then walked to the bathroom with an empty cheese bag. I asked him where he was going with the bag. He said he didn't know. He walked back into the kitchen and put the empty bag in the refrigerator drawer. He seemed very disoriented as to where he was.

July 6

I took him to another appointment today at the Brain Center. No change in meds at this time. Beecher has gotten clumsier lately because of reduced judgment. Dr. Léger noted that Beecher was participating in regular exercise several times a week.

He has also recently developed an interest in watercolor and has produced stunning works. His new found interest in art is unusual, but has been described in certain patients with FTD. The doctor asked if he could obtain copies of some of Beecher's work, which I agreed to. His diagnosis is now Frontotemporal dementia with behavioral disturbance or bvFTD.

Simple things are not so simple any more for him; he is losing common sense. While I was busy painting, I heard him banging on something in the other room.

I walked into the dining room to find a picture on my glass dining room table. He had been trying to nail a hanger on it to give to a friend at Day Care. The nail was too big. I got a smaller one and told him not to do it on that table as he could break the glass.

I carried it into the other room and then I noticed he had a large knife and that he was carrying the blade part in his hand and had been using the handle as a hammer. I took it away from him and gave him a hammer.

July 27-30

Yay, a three-day weekend getaway with my daughters to Newport Beach, CA.! Awesome time! Dining at our favorite places, beach time, bike riding on the boardwalk, ferry to Balboa Island, frozen bananas and fantastic weather! My son in law, Cole, Michelle's husband, watched Beecher for me at their home. He was pretty good. Just got a little anxiety but overall did well. I knew he was in good hands with Cole.

August 5

Amy picked Beecher up and took him to the movies and lunch. They stopped at the 99cent store for candy. He walked in and stood in line at the register. She told him to go get the candy first. He went and got the candy and then started to walk out without paying for it. On the way home after the movies, he did the same thing at Vons when they went in to get some tea. A week later, he and I went into the 99cent store. He started putting soda in a hand carrying basket. I told him we needed the bigger shopping cart and I walked outside the store to get one and told him to wait for me. As I was getting the cart, he walked outside the store with the soda in his hands and put them in the cart and then went back inside the store. Everything is so out of sorts. There are no more filters for him to do normal things.

August 9

I got a letter from Harry Reid's office in regards to the letter I sent in May. His office will get in contact with me once they have an answer for me.

August 16

One of Beecher's friends asked him on Facebook how he was doing. This was his response: *"I am doing fine Robert I have Picks disease it's frontotemporal lobar degeneration my frontal lobes are misfiring I am having problems with my speech and other cognitive functions."* It's amazing that he got all the words spelled correctly but he made it all into one sentence!

August 18

My sister, Patti picked us up to take us to the movies. The next day, I had gone to dance class and when I got home, Beecher said he couldn't find his wallet. I told him we would find it later. I figured it would be in the house somewhere as he had it when we went to dance class that day and we had not left the house since. For a week I searched every possible place I thought it would be and I was ready to order new I.D. card and insurance cards. A week later Patti called and said she found his wallet in the back seat near where he had been sitting when we went to the movies. That means he had the wallet on him the whole time and must have taken it out of his pocket and laid it on the seat. Also, today I had to repair the toilet as he could not figure out how to do it.

August 31

Guess I got too lazy or too busy to post during the remainder of the month, so here is a summary of the month. During the month of August, he has fallen four times; twice in the closet, once coming out of the bedroom and once in the kitchen. No injuries except he hurt his elbow in the closet.

This month so far, he has broken a dish of mine that I had for 50 years, the handle on the toilet, a glass and I don't know how many other things I have yet to find broken or missing.

Sometimes he puts his dress shirts in the drawer and hangs up the t-shirts. He can't make gravy anymore; it used to be his specialty. Many times, when I ask him why he did something, he doesn't give me an explanation. He just repeats what it was that he did over and over. For example, I ask, "Why did you throw that in the sink and not the garbage disposal?" He says, "I threw it in the sink" every time I ask.

This month has been very trying as he is getting harder and harder to communicate with him. His attention span is much worse. When he talks to me, he stares at my chest if I am standing and he is sitting down. He won't look me in the eyes. Seems to zone out a lot when I'm talking to him. Won't follow my commands. I have to tell him sometimes four or five times and he just gets a glazed look on his face and goes back to what he was doing.

When his friend came over to pick him up to take him to dinner and a meeting, he didn't acknowledge him for at least a minute or so. He was too absorbed in his iPad and even then, he just got up and went to put his shoes on.

He often turns the light off when I'm in the bathroom and most of the time doesn't turn it off when he leaves the room (any room). He closes doors on me.

One day, after shopping as we were putting groceries in the trunk of my car, he started to close the trunk while I was still putting groceries in it. I asked him to stop twice. But he continued and slammed the trunk down on my arm. I started yelling at him and he just turned around and went to get in the car. I'm sure many shoppers thought I was a maniac.

As I was getting something out of the fridge one day, he walked over to get something out and closed the door on me. He has no sense of who he might bump into with the cart in the store. Several times he almost ran into children.

Sometimes he talks to me and tells me things like; I have frontotemporal dementia, as if I am someone else. I'm embarrassed to say that several times, I said, "That's no excuse for everything." Sometimes I just can't take much more of this and I always regret it after I say it.

Seems very confused a lot but always remembers things that matter to him, in regards to day care or painting a picture for someone. Obsessive behaviors are worse than ever.

He picks his teeth constantly, uses a lot of baby wipes, eats a lot of Tums and always wants more Probiotics and fiber pills in addition to yogurt. Still continues to empty dishwasher as soon as it runs its cycle instead of waiting for it to dry. Washes clothes every other day. Still does dishes, but makes a bigger mess.

I had to finally tell him not to do the pans as he doesn't clean well and makes more work for me. Brushes his teeth excessively and also uses mouthwash ten or more times a day.

I don't know who this person is anymore. I can no longer relate to him. He's not the person I married 23 years ago. I'm lonely and I miss my husband, not this one. I'm sure someone came in and stole his brain and just lives here for me to take care of. FTD not only robs you of your loved one but it is a soul snatcher and I'm starting to hate it more and more each day. The man I married has literally disappeared in front of my eyes. I grieve daily for both of us. I recently read somewhere that it's okay to cry and to remember that tears are prayers too and they travel to God when we can't speak. I have many days when I choke up trying to hold back the tears.

Came home from class and he told me he couldn't find his iPad. Spent two hours looking for it as I knew it had to be in the house somewhere; even checked the trash cans, because two days before I found his sunglasses in the outside recycled bin when I went to put out trash. Thought about what he had done while I was gone and remember he had washed his clothes which he puts on bed after taking out of dryer. I had already looked under bed and around bed. Dawned on me it might be in between the end of the bed and foot board. And there it was; can't believe it hadn't fallen through!

**I think I'm somewhere between giving up and seeing how much more I can take! That just about sums it up!**

September 3

Beecher was on the toilet eating yogurt; came into the kitchen with the empty yogurt and spoon in one hand and his underwear in the other. He rinsed off the spoon and laid the underwear on the kitchen counter. Started walking to the other bathroom with the spoon and left the underwear on counter.

TV habits; has a lot of programs saved on DVR. He will watch one almost to the end, say the last five to ten minutes and then switches to another show. Doesn't bother to delete the one he was watching. Also, when we are watching one of our favorite shows, he will do searches for other shows. Sometimes he will delete a show that I haven't watched right after I tell him not to delete it, he will delete anyway. I cry everyday either in the shower or in bed after he has gone to sleep. I don't want him to hear me cry. The meltdowns are coming more and more often and I sometimes think I'll go crazy. I try to keep up the smiley face and laughter, but I realize that when I'm scared inside, I joke to keep from being afraid and losing my sanity.

September 5

Received a letter from the office of Congressman Joe Heck in regards to the letter I sent to Harry Reid. A case officer was assigned to my case to give me an update. In communicating with Harry Reid's office, they came to the same conclusion. He stated that when it comes to changing VA laws, the body that does this is the House of Veterans Affairs Committee and the Senate Veteran Affairs Committee. That is where changes to VA laws must pass. Once it passes out of those committees, the Congressman and other members of Congress who are not in the VA committee can finally vote "yay" or "nay" on the proposed VA law. As of now, they need nothing from me.

Note: As of August 2019, I have never gotten any other response. In

2015, I also wrote a letter to Dina Titus, Nevada U.S. Representative and never got an answer back.

~

September 19

Appointment with Dr. Léger at the Brain Center. Beecher is now seeing Dr. Léger every six months. Since his last visit Beecher has had some motor difficulties. He has had several falls probably due to coordination. When he gets off balance, he doesn't have the ability to right himself before falling. Dr. Léger said he also has some Parkinsonism's. Beecher also sometimes chokes on food probably because he tries to eat too quickly. Dr. Léger suggested I make an appointment at the VA to have a swallow evaluation done. I brought in all of his watercolors that Dr. Léger had asked for. He said he would make copies and put them on a flash drive and return them to me. He said Beecher's speech is soft and difficult to hear and that he has an intense stare with reduced blinking. Beecher had also been on the med Seroquel but now Dr. Léger wants to replace it with Mirtazapine. That should help with sleep and obsessive behaviors. He wants Beecher to go off the Trazodone. He has been taking three tabs each night for a total of 300 mg. Sometime in the near future they want to start him on a new drug called Nuedexta. They have now added a secondary diagnosis of Corticobasal Syndrome. Also Dr. Léger recommended a Physical Rehabilitation and Sports Therapy session here at the Brain Center. Someone will call me to set up.

~

September 26

I took Beecher to the VA for a swallow test. The test was inconclusive as to indicate a serious problem.

~

October 5

Beecher's birthday was on October 2 and to celebrate, Amy and her boyfriend took us to the Adventure Dome at Circus, Circus which included lots of rides which Beecher loved and he spent the evening smiling a lot and also going to the bathroom a lot! He also managed to get lost several times but we found him! He's such a kid at heart!

∽

October 11

We drove down to Laughlin to attend Beecher's nephew's wedding. His nephew, Tyler was getting married at one of the casinos. Beecher was not at all social and pretty much stayed away from everyone to avoid having to talk to anyone except for his nephews a couple of times.

They hadn't seen him lately and didn't realize how much he had changed. After the ceremony and after eating mostly cake and candy, Beecher disappeared. We couldn't find him.

As we had booked a one-night stay at the Hotel/Casino where the couple got married, I went to look for him. I asked several people if they had seen him.

It turned out he had gone down to the elevator, and was looking for our room and had gotten off on the wrong floor. I finally found him and called it a night.

∽

October 13

The next Grant got approved for Adult Day Care. This one was from Helping Hands and was for $1000 which was for fourteen weeks!

∽

October 15

It's my birthday. Doesn't feel like it except I think I've aged twice as much these last two years. If I could have one wish, I'd wish this disease would just disappear from our lives. Frances bought two cards for me from Beecher and let him choose which one he wanted to give me. She helped him sign the card. He handed it to me and seemed very pleased. Made me cry. Frances is so very thoughtful. I am blessed to have her as our caregiver, but she is more than that. She is an amazing person and now a true friend. I couldn't do all this without her. Amy took me to dinner at a Mediterranean Lounge and the next day I drove to Pahrump to have lunch with my two best friends from high school, Sandy and Judy, to celebrate our birthdays. Frances watched Beecher. Thank goodness for family, friends and Frances!

~

November 25-30

My sister Patti invited us to go on a trip to Northern California for Thanksgiving where my other sister Linda and my brother Donny live. The drive went fairly well, except for the time Beecher got out of the car at the gas station to go to the bathroom and banged the car door against the pillar by the pumps, putting a dent in Patti's fairly new car. Once we arrived, Beecher pretty much kept to himself playing with his iPad. My niece and her three boys came over Thanksgiving Day along with my brother and his wife. My nephews loved Beecher. They were always on his lap and liked watching him play Angry Birds. He was like another kid in the room. When they came over the next day, the first thing the youngest one said was, "Where is that guy that I like?"

One day we drove to Lake Tahoe for the day. While walking on the rocks where people build "art rocks" Beecher fell and hurt his elbow. Good thing my brother-in-law is a doctor. He helped Beecher up and he seemed to be okay. The last night we were there he fell in the bedroom during the night. It woke me up but he said he was okay. Two days after we got home, he showed me his elbow which was swollen as big as a mandarin orange from the fall on the rocks. Also, my sister called after we got home and said that when he fell the night before we left, he had knocked the closet door off the hinge. Nobody had noticed before we left. I ended up taking Beecher to his primary doctor to look at his elbow but there were no broken bones just swelling. He kept an ace bandage on it for several days until he wrapped it too tight one day and I had to take him to quick care because he had cut off the circulation. He almost had to have his wedding ring cut off, but I got him home in enough of time and used soap to take it off. Never put the ring back on after that. That was sad, but I couldn't take a chance and with the added weight on him it was already tight anyway. And later it would be too loose when he lost weight.

❧

December 5

He put jelly over scrambled eggs. That was a new one!

❧

December 13

I decided to take him to our annual Christmas party at our clubhouse. He started getting ready three hours early. Nanny Franny put his belt in his pants and laid them on the bed. He told her, "Take out the belt, right now!" He repeated it twice and then said, "I don't wear belts." She went into clean the bathroom and he came in and turned down the bed and started getting undressed. He said he was going to bed. She told him it wasn't time for bed. He was going to a party in a few hours. He did good at the party and after he ate dinner, he actually danced a few dances with me to my surprise. It was a short night but fun.

❧

December 14

I decided to take him to a Holiday party at our friend's house from our dance class. Tonight, he put the belt on his pants! He was very unsociable and wanted to go home as soon as he had eaten. He was very sloppy and dripping food wherever he walked. After he got some coffee and almost dropped the coffee cup, I decided it was time to go home. This had to be his last party. I couldn't continue to do this to the hostesses. They were very understanding as they know Beecher and he had been attending dance classes with me for over a year. I apologized to our hostess and took him home.

December 16

Amy's band BET was performing at Vinyl at The Hard Rock. All of the family went. We all loved it including Beecher. The only problem was he kept getting up every few minutes to go to the bathroom. I finally told him to quit getting up and down as he was annoying the other people and he finally stopped. I don't know why he does this, but it happens every time we go to the movies as well. He usually stops going once the movie starts, but on the way into the theatre, he stops at every bathroom. Must be some anxiety thing.

December 19

Before leaving for day care Beecher was sitting in his recliner. All of a sudden, he said, "Suzanne gave me a blow job in the bathroom." I said, "She did?' He said "No just kidding." A few minutes later he said, "It didn't happen." He wouldn't answer me when I asked him if it did or it didn't happen. I don't know what to believe anymore and does it really even matter?

~

December 24

I invited the family and a few friends over for Christmas Eve at our house. Beecher liked dressing up with his Santa hat. I had the feeling this might be the last Christmas Eve at our home. His symptoms were getting worse, and I was looking into a home for him in the near future. He was having way too many falls and it was becoming a safety issue for both of us.

~

December 25

Christmas Day–We went to dinner at my grandson's house. Nice time, except for following him around to clean up his spills. Beecher had painted a really cute Christmas card with a snowman and animals on it. I painted one with a picture of dogs driving a truck. Everyone loved it!

Note: Sometime during the early part of this year, I don't remember when, but he became obsessed with the idea of going to Brazil to visit John of God whom he thought would heal him. He had a friend that he had met at his meditation meetings last year that was trying to talk him into going. I explained that we had no money to go and the trip alone was several thousand dollars each, not to mention the boarding at a remote village for both of us. Even if we had the money for him, I could not just let him go by himself! He would not let up about the subject and he honestly didn't understand when I explained to him that if it was true that he could be healed that everyone would be going to Brazil. I feel so sorry for him as I know he is desperate, but I couldn't concede to him going.

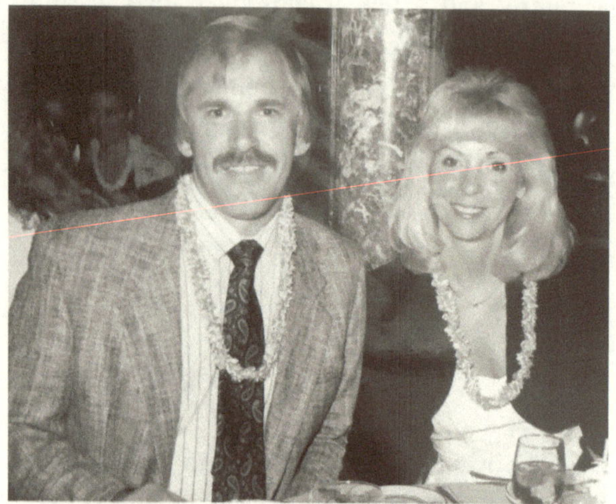

Beecher & I met in November 1988. He was a member of the Elks Lodge #1468 and we spent a lot of time there over the years. In March 1991 we went on our very first cruise to the Mexican Rivera with 6 other couples from the Elks Lodge.

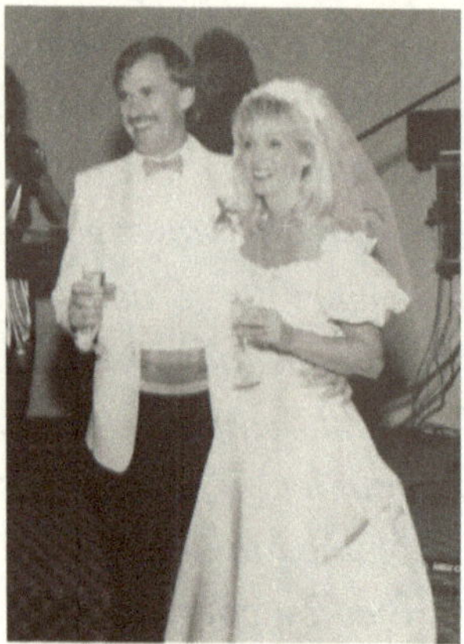

Our Wedding Day – June 15, 1991. We were the 1st couple to get married at this lodge.

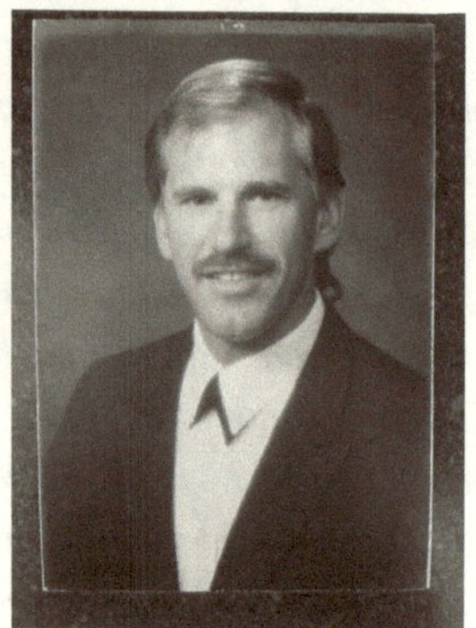

Beecher became the Exalted Ruler of Elks Lodge #1468 from 1995-1996. By the time of his death, he had been a member for 30 years.

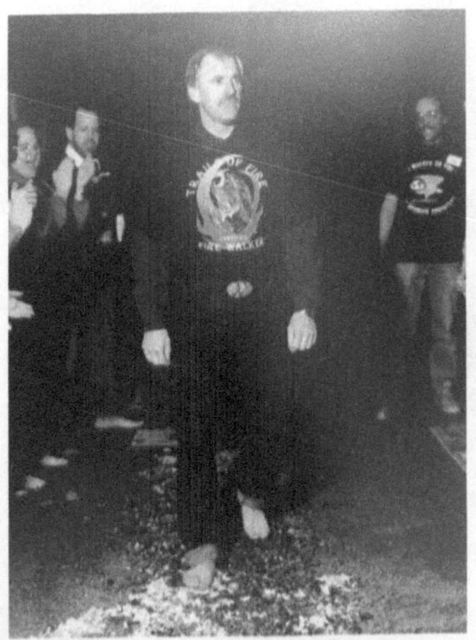

Firewalking! What a thrill!" If you've never tried it, you are missing a great experience! Beecher & I became Certified Fire Walk Instructors & we taught our "Trails of Fire" course for over 5 years on a monthly basis until we got burned out. NO pun intended!

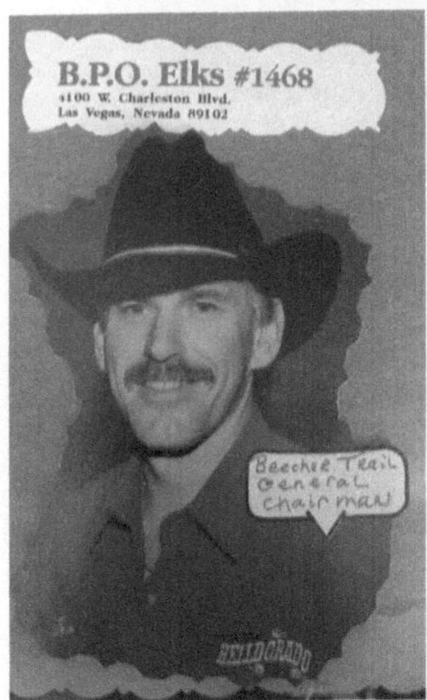

Beecher was also General Chairman of Helldorado in 1996.

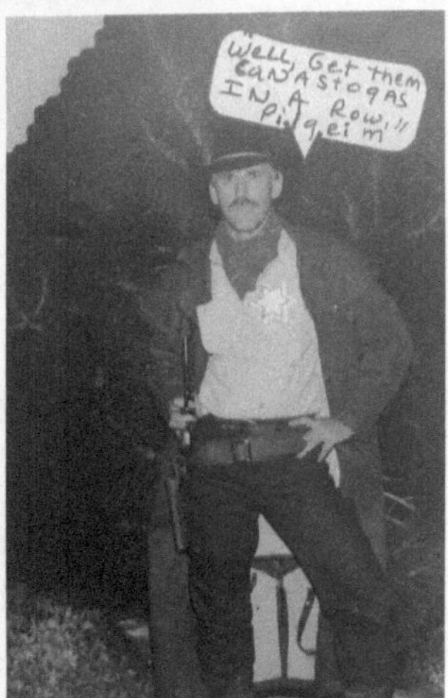

Helldorado Ranger 1996. "Well, put them Canastoga's in a circle, Pilgrim!" Beecher was a man of many voices and he loved to imitate John Wayne.

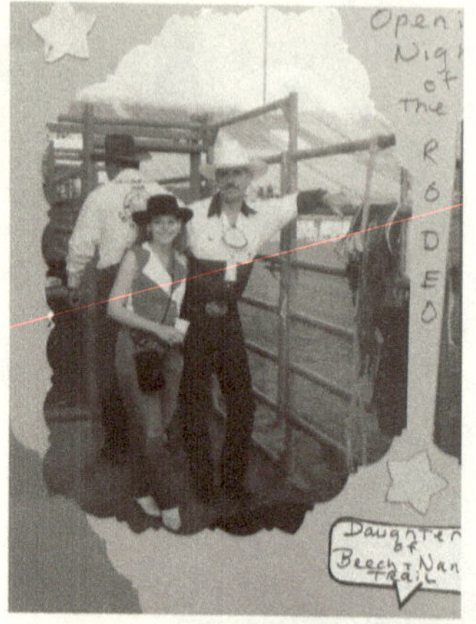

Beecher & Amy at the Helldorado Rodeo in 1996. Amy sang "The Star Spangled Banner." We were all so proud of her, especially Beecher.

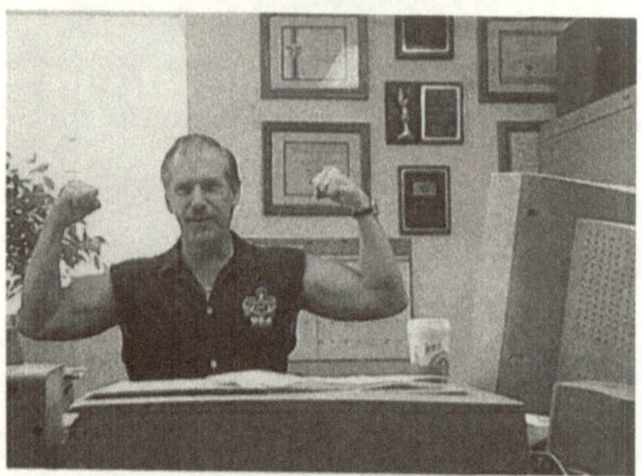

Beecher was a martial artist in many types of styles. He earned a brown belt in Taekwondo in 1998. He loved to show off his big guns!

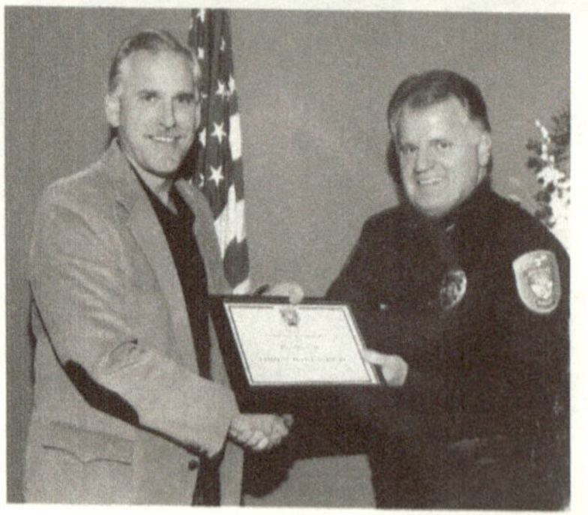

In 2002, Beecher attended a "ride along" program with Las Vegas Police and was awarded "Police Citizens Academy Certificate."

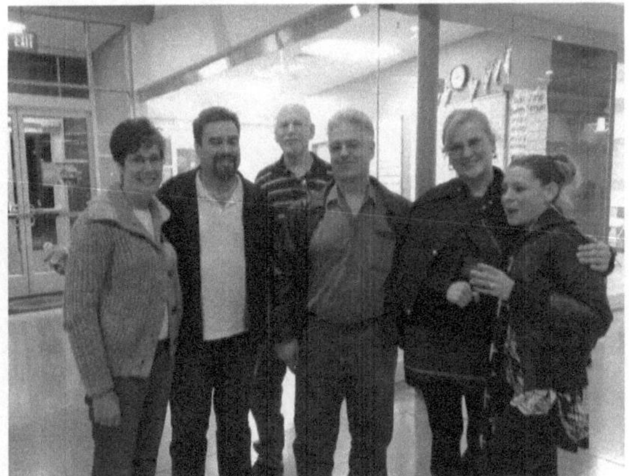

On January 20, 2014, our watercolor teacher entered us into a Fine Art Show at the Multigenerational Center for a one night showing. Beecher was so excited. My daughter Amy and several of our friends, Paul & Debbie and Jimmy & Kathy attended. He loved showing off his work.

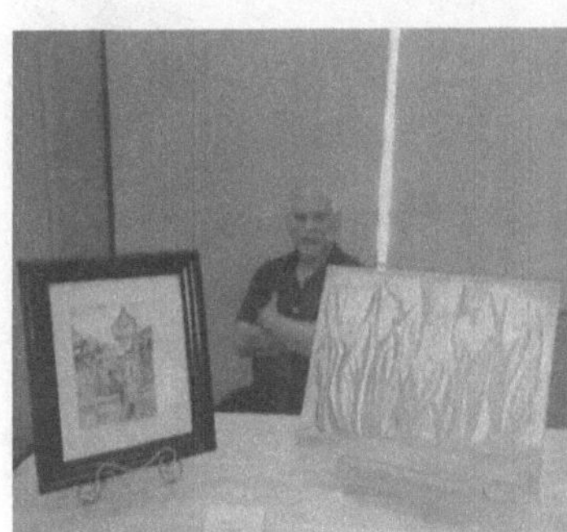

June 1, 2014. Another Fine Art Show at the Community Center at Solera where we lived. Beecher entered 2 painting. He was really excited especially because one lady bought one of his paintings!

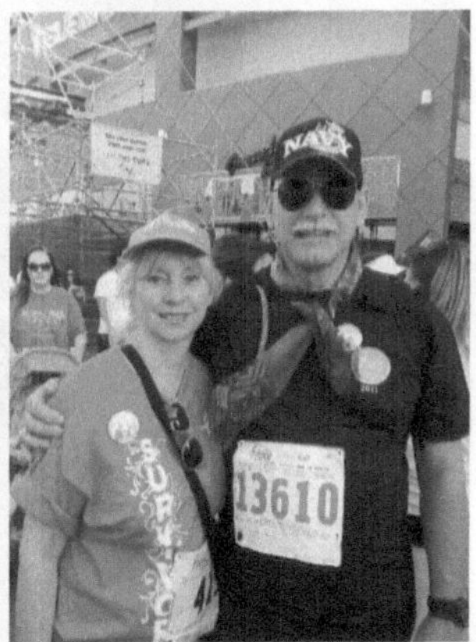

Beecher joined me in the "Race for the Cure on May 7, 2011. I was 1 year cancer free! Some facial expressions were starting to show up but we didn't know anything serious was going on with him. He was proud to wear his Navy Seabee's hat as he was a Veteran during the Vietnam War.

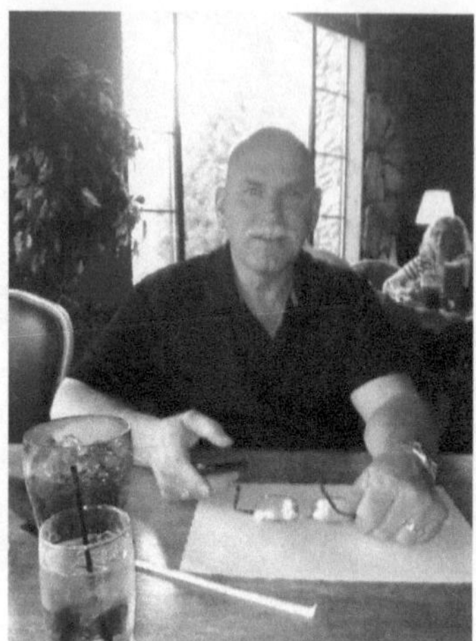

Our 22st Anniversary at Mt. Charleston Hotel 6-15-13.

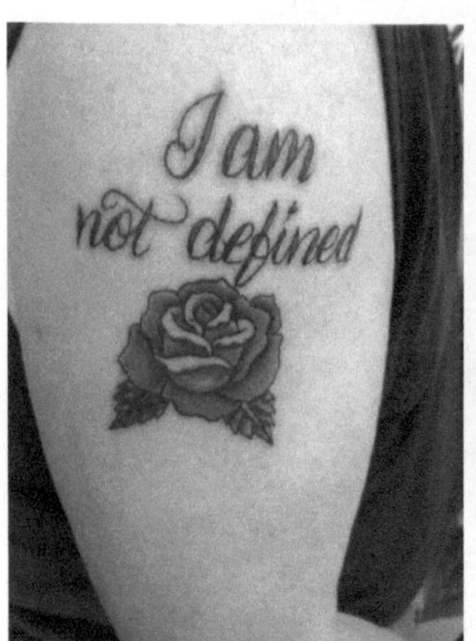

Beecher's 1st and only Tattoo that he had done on 7-13-13. "I am not defined." Beecher believed that you should not give up defining yourself to others and to not be concerned with how others define you. He is not defined by his illness but by the great things he has done in his life.

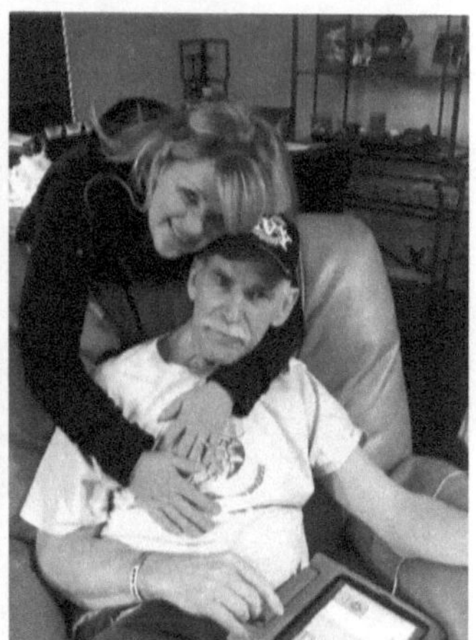

Michelle & Beecher 10-18-13. This picture was taken shortly after Beecher had been diagnosed with Frontotemporal Dementia (FTD). The facial expressions and the loss of weight says a lot of what was happening to him.

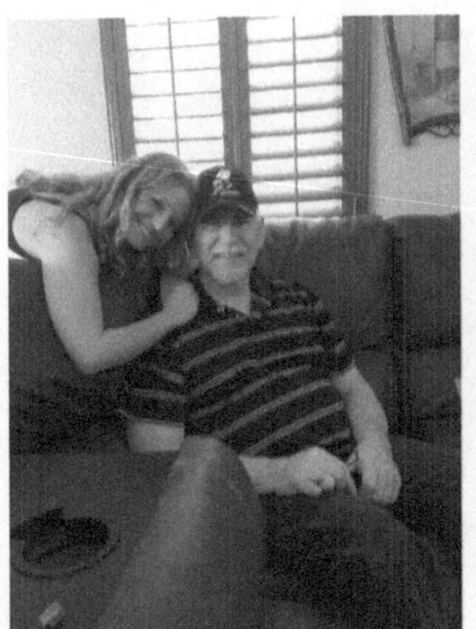

Beecher & Amy @Michelle's & Coles house in the summer of 2014 before we went to Newport Beach, CA. July 27-30 for a Mommy and daughters getaway. Beecher stayed with Cole.

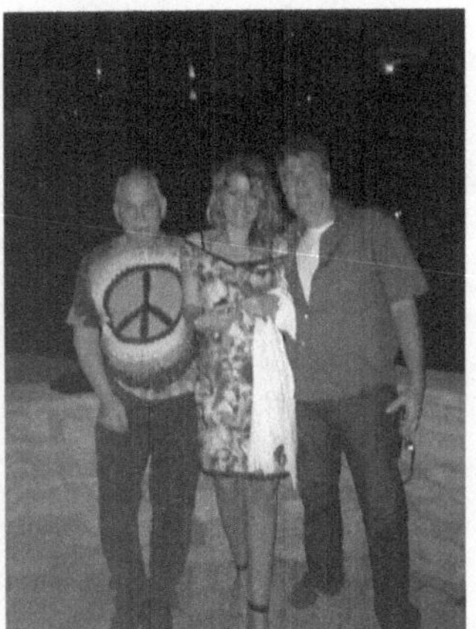

We drove to Lake Las Vegas in April 2015 with our friend Gary and his girlfriend shortly before Beecher went to live in a Memory Care home. We had a great time even though Beecher wandered away several time but we eventually found him! Gary was surprised how much Beecher had declined since the last time he saw him.

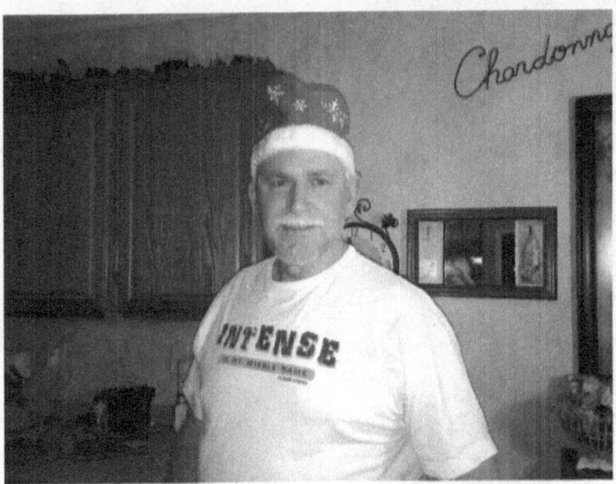

Beecher loved to wear hats and he had many of them. Here he is in one of his Christmas hats in 2013.

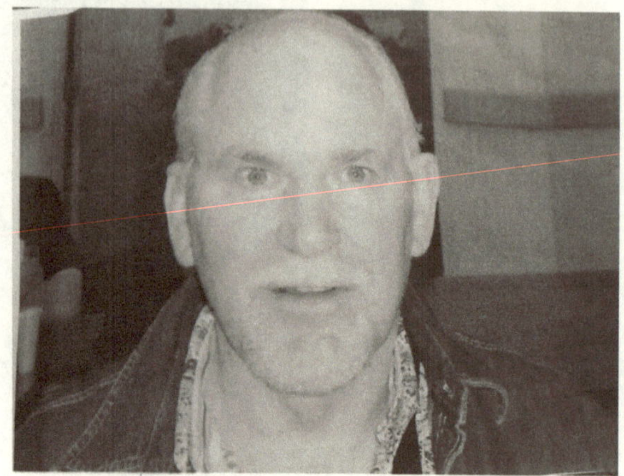

One of the signs of FTD is the glassy look in the eyes.
This is very apparent in this picture in 2015.

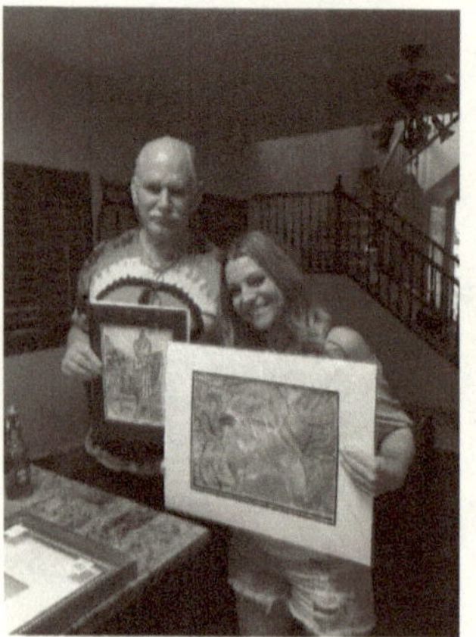

Beecher's gift to Amy on her 38th birthday were
2 copies of his favorite paintings, "Time" and
"Colorful Bird."

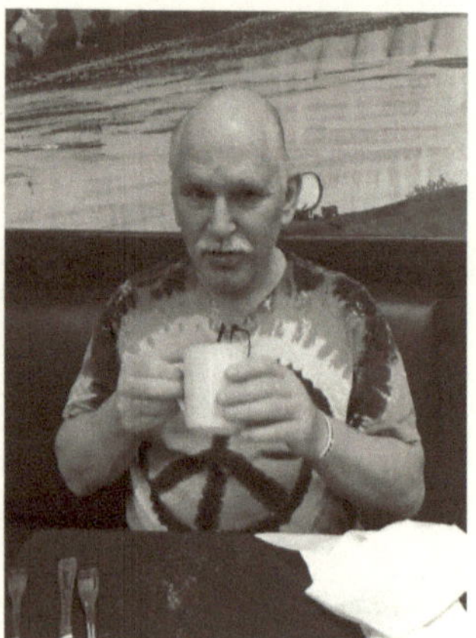

Took Beecher out to our last breakfast together at
Egg Works before moving to the home he will
live in from now on.

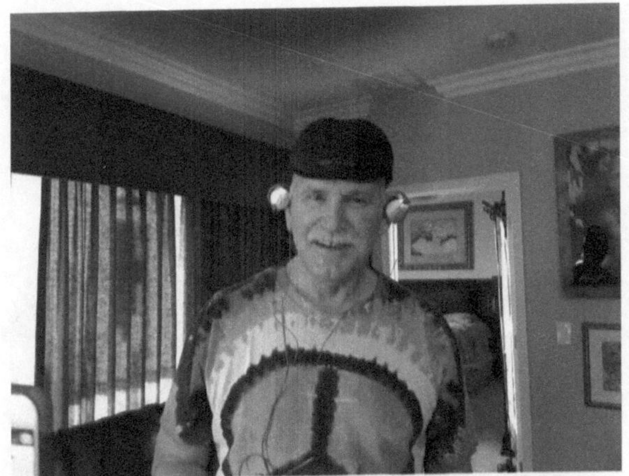

Beecher with his headphones. The night before he moved to his new home, he walked out of the bedroom with his headphones on, but sticking out of instead of in his ears. We all got a good laugh out it including him when he realized we were laughing at him.

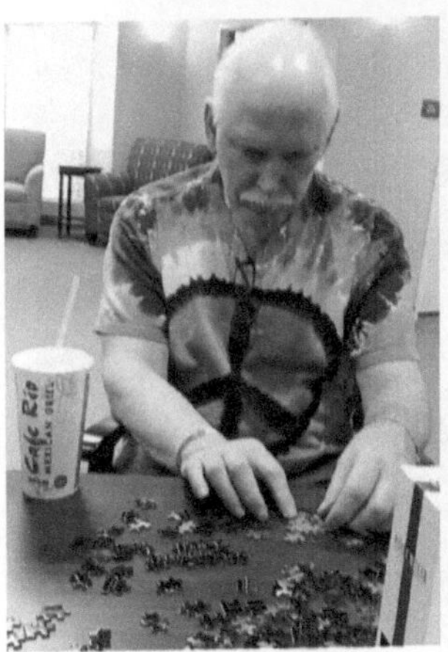

Beecher spends a lot of time in the facility putting together puzzles. By the way, do you notice he has his tie-dyed t-shirt on again? It was his favorite shirt of all time.

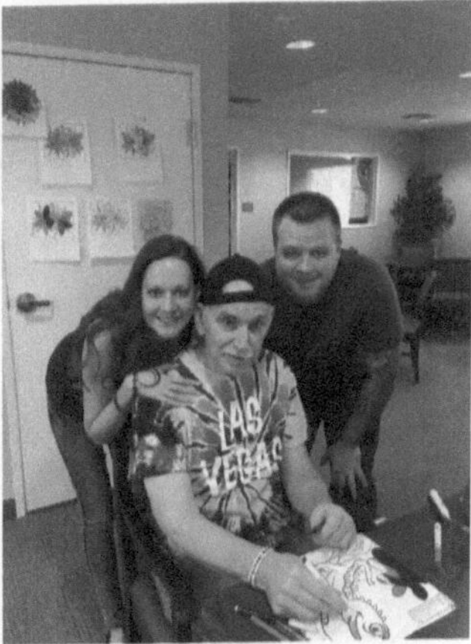

My grandson Justin and his wife Bethany came to visit him at the facility. He was very excited to see them.

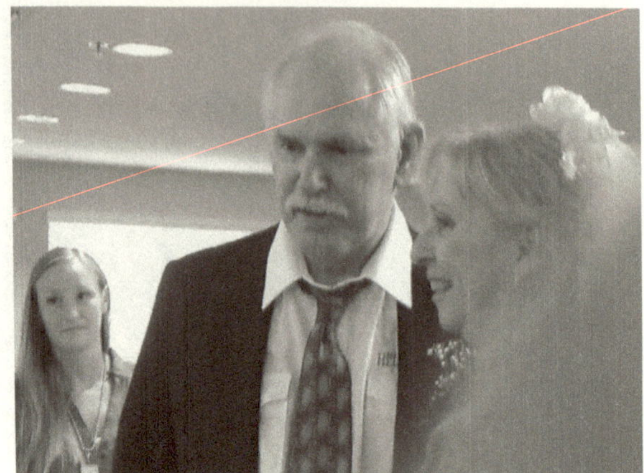

We renewed our vows for the third time at the memory care facility on our 24th Wedding Anniversary, June 15, 2015. We renewed our vows for the 2nd time in 1995 walking over hot coals! (Now that was a hot time in the old town that night!)

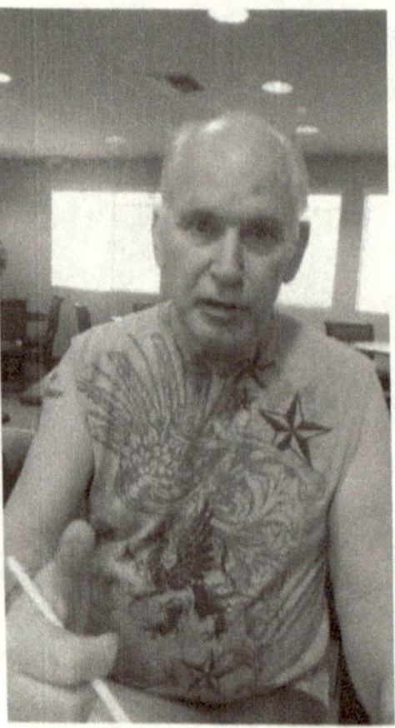

Beecher spent most of his time at the facility, coloring and doing puzzles. He had slowed down doing watercolor because he had a hard time holding the brushes to paint.

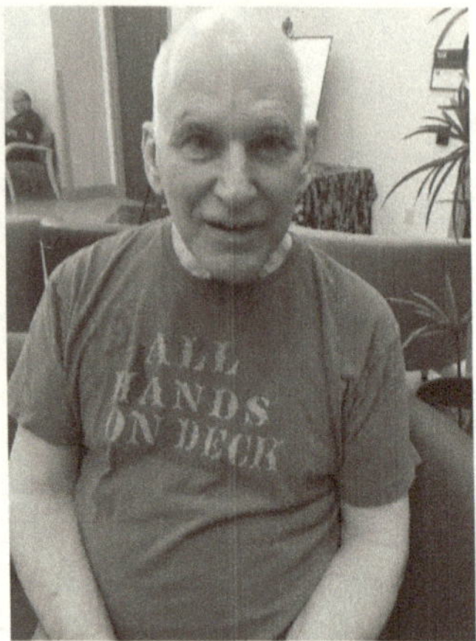

Beecher's friend Glenn came to visit him and give him a massage. Boy did he like that, as you can tell from the smile on his face!

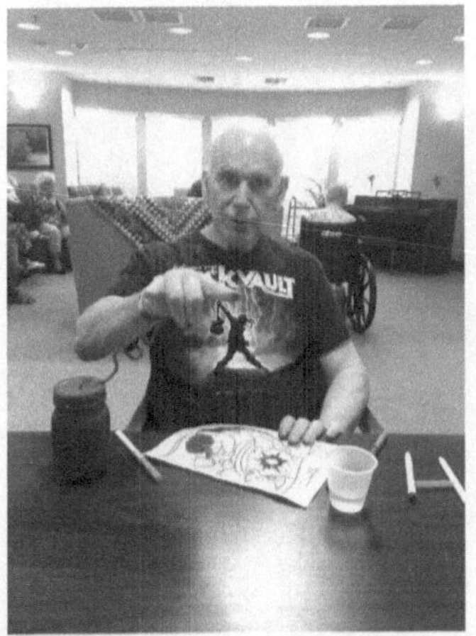

At this time, Beecher is starting to lose a lot of weight and his facial expressions are much the same and he is unrecognizable to most of his friends. With FDT, his memory is intact, but the disease has started taking away more and more of his personality and the man he was. It was devasting to watch. Some of his friends that came to visit included Janon & Kent, Kim & Steve and Mike & JoAnn, the girls from dance class and our watercolor class.

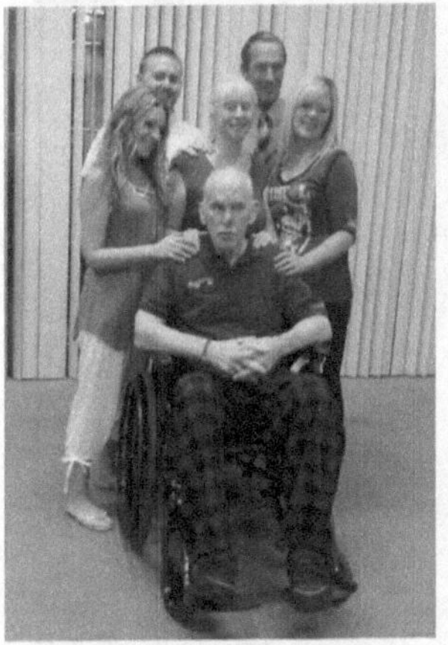

The Elks Lodge put on a Pot Luck Benefit to raise money for us. There was a nice turnout and an overflow of love. So thankful to have so many loving friends and family. Pictured are Amy, my grandson Tyler, myself, my son-in-law Cole, and Michelle.

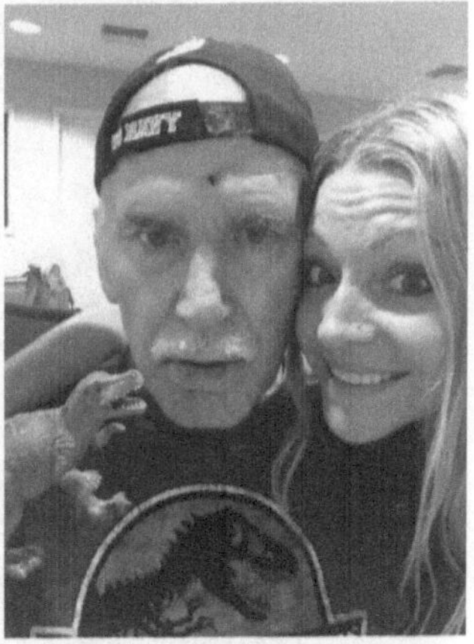

We had a birthday party for Beecher's 61st birthday, Oct 2, 2015. Amy brought Jurassic Park decorations since the newest 2015 Jurassic World movie just came out and Beecher loved the movie.

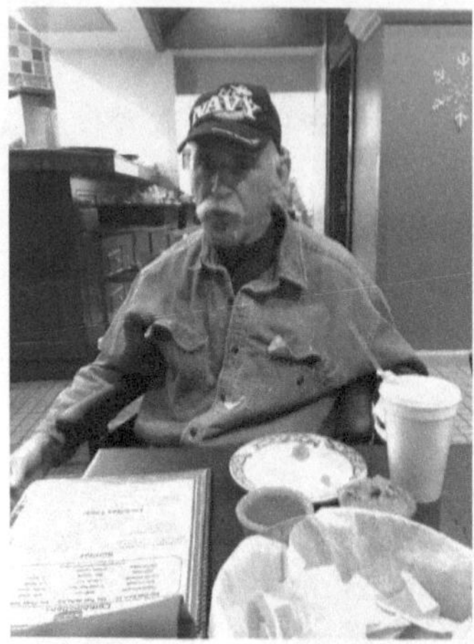

Amy & I took Beecher to Sam's Town to the Christmas Laser Show at Sam's Town. Beecher has been in a wheelchair for awhile now. He was fascinated by the lights. We ate some dinner and then went over to Roxy's Lounge where Beecher had proposed to me 26 years ago. It was a fun and sentimental evening.

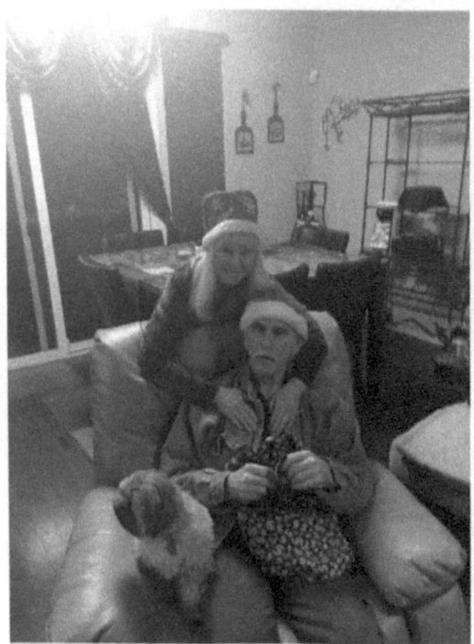

Christmas dinner 2015 at Michelle & Coles house.
We both have our Christmas hats on!

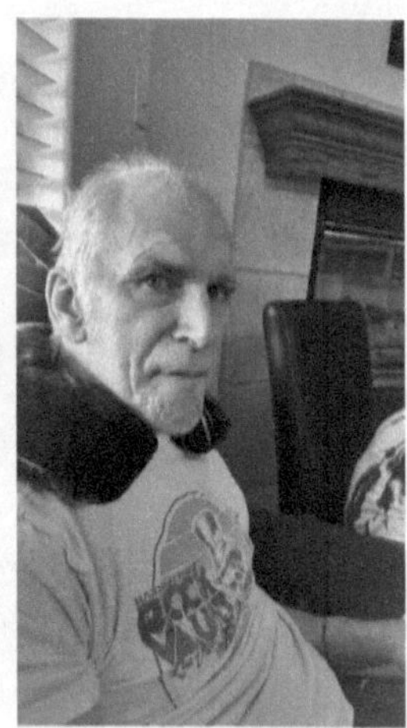

Beecher's not happy about something.
He looks like he has aged 10 years.

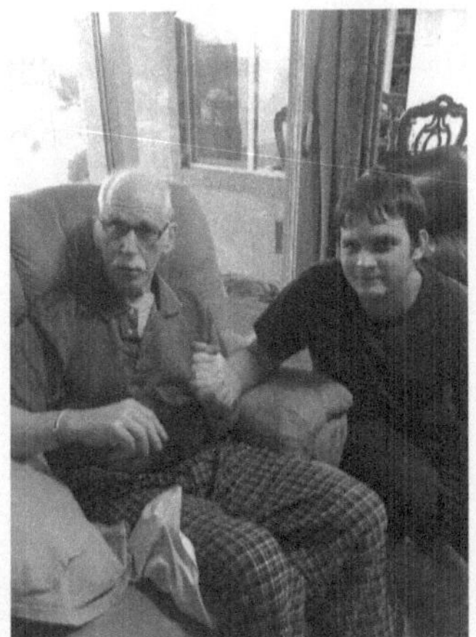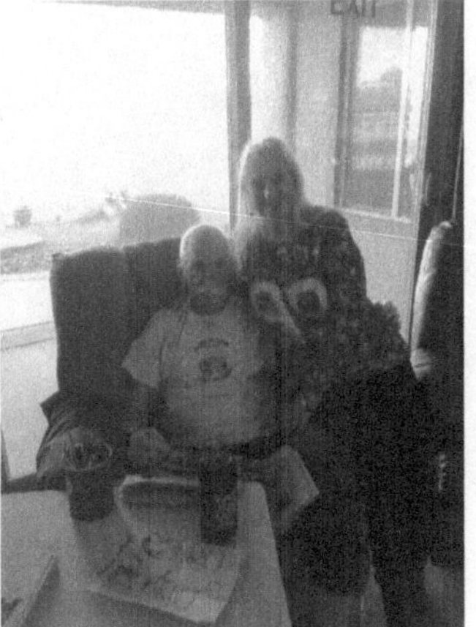

Our grandson Zech came to visit Beech at his 2nd
home on 12-30-15. He had not seen him in awhile
and was very sad to see his Grandpa look so different. But we had a nice visit with him.

Another visit with Beecher at the 2nd home. He
seems so quiet and sad but we had a nice time. He
is the only patient at this home.
I'm sure he must be very lonely.

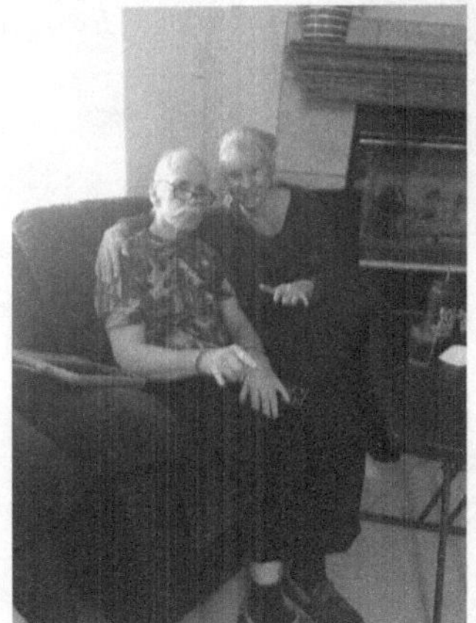

On January 1, 2016 I had to move Beecher to another home because their caregiver
moved! This is his 3rd home now. I'm sure he is just about as tired as I am with all
the moves! But this home turns out to be the best one of all! One of the caregivers
took this picture of us giving each other the I Love You sign in sign language.

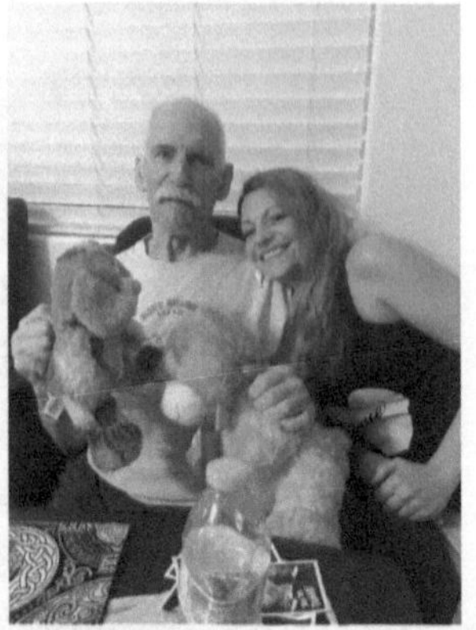

Valentine's Day with Beecher and Amy. One of his favorite days. He loved the stuffed animals and the Peeps candy (his favorite). He was in a happy mood. I think he likes the new home.
Great caregivers!

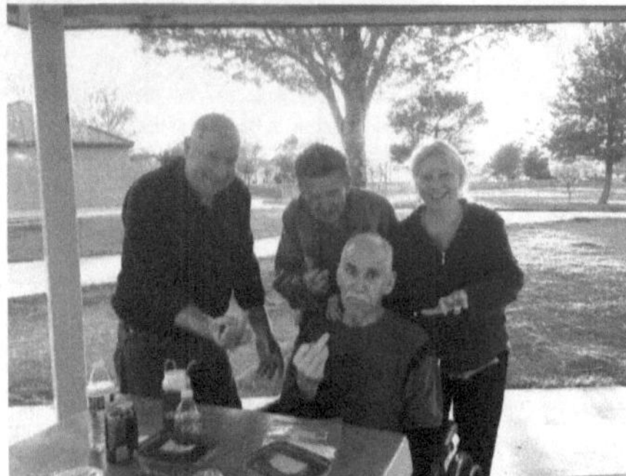

This was the funniest day with Beecher's friends visiting from Arizona. Beecher was trying to give his friends "the I love you" sign but his fingers wouldn't work so I said. "Why don't you give Gary the finger instead and he did!" His friend Gary said "He does remember me." We all laughed so hard including Beecher who got a big kick out of it too. The look on his face was priceless!"

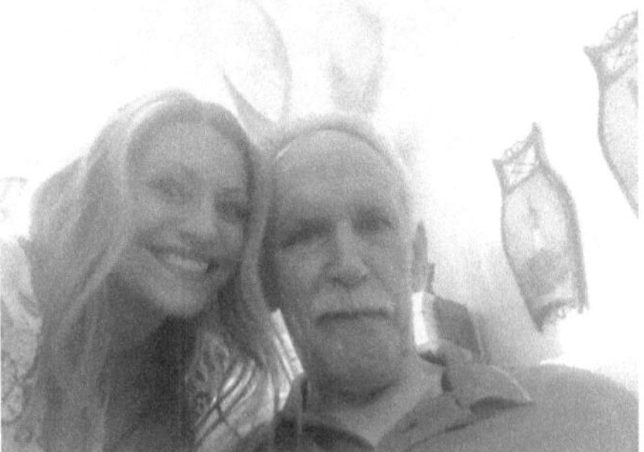

Beecher loves Easter! He likes to wear the bunny ears!

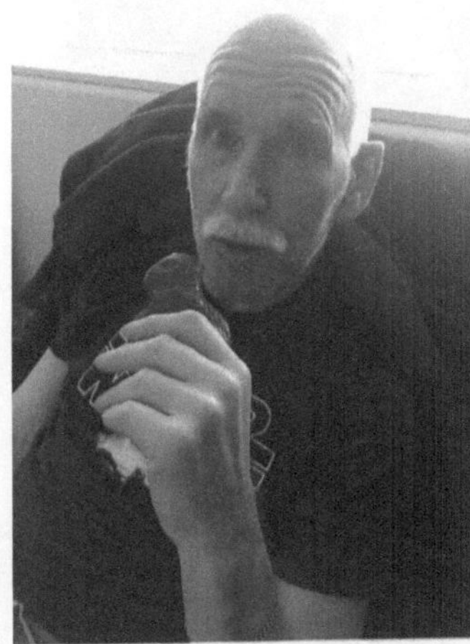

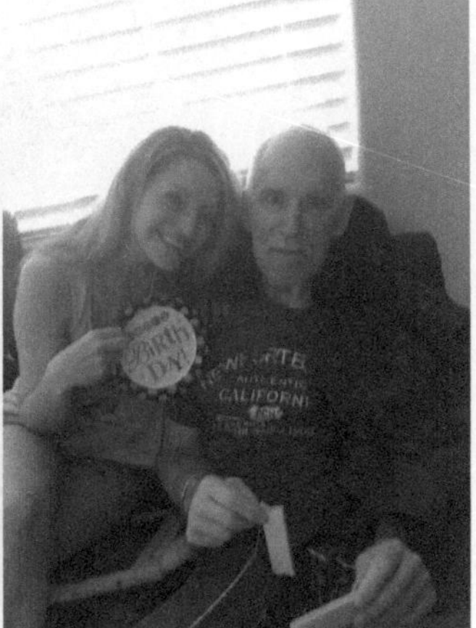

But mostly he likes the Chocolate Easter Bunny! We're starting to see a quick decline in Beecher as this disease starts taking on more rapidly. This is the ugliness of this horrible devastating disease. I hate what it has done to him.

We celebrated Amy's 39th Birthday on May 2, 2016. Beecher got a kick out of spanking her!

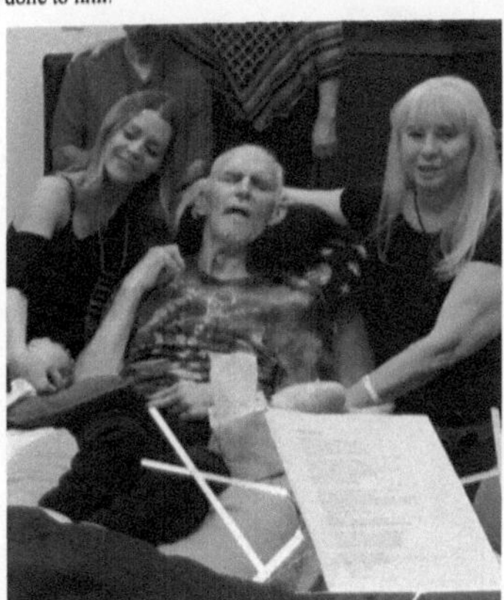

This picture was taken 3 days before he passed. We were celebrating our October birthdays at the home. A lot of friends and performers attended and sang some of our favorite songs. Although he seemed somewhat uncomfortable at times, he did seem to enjoy the music. Also, the other residents and caregivers got to see a live show and they really enjoyed it!

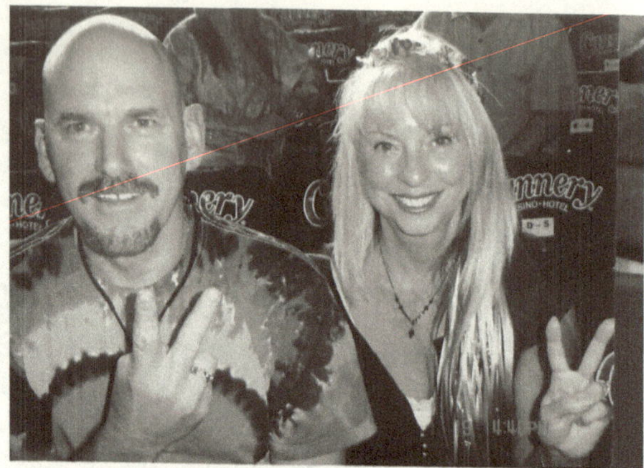

These are the days I want to remember him most. Full of life and the music he loved so much at the Cannery Hotel in North Las Vegas. Many good times were spent there for years at the concerts such as - Bobby Vee, Johnny Tillotson, Gene Pitney, The Lovin Spoonful, Blood, Sweat & Tears, Glen Fry (founding member of The Eagles), Ambrosia, Gary Wright, John Ford Coley, Steven Bishop, and Cannery Stock (a mini Woodstock!) with a Jimmy Hendricks Tribute and the original lead singer of Santana (Greg Rolie) and last but not least, The Guess Who! Beecher you will be remembered! You know my saying, Life's a Beech, and then you marry one! I hope your dancing in the sky!

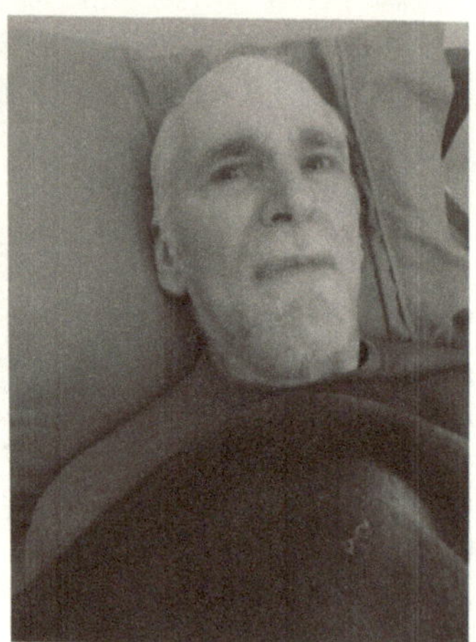

The last goodbye.

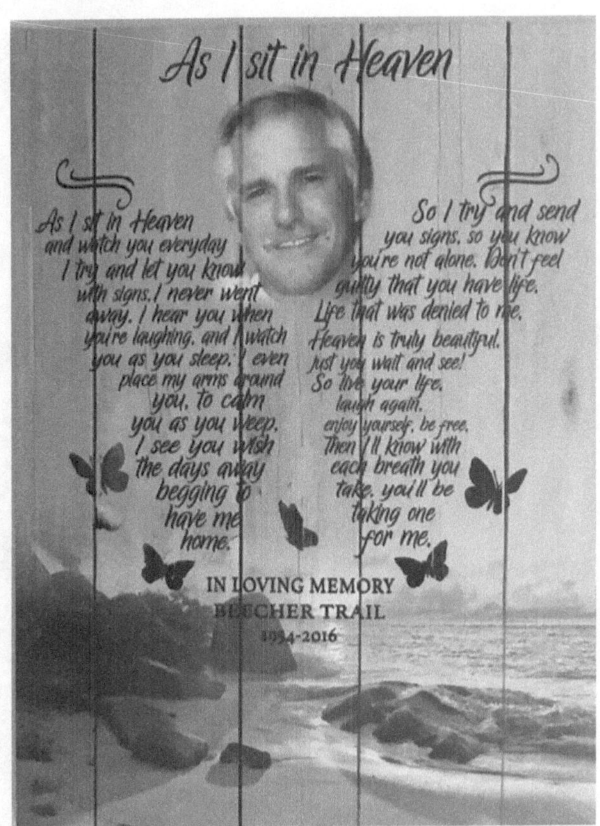

In Memory of Beecher Trail or "Beech" as most people called him.

CHAPTER 5

2015—THE YEAR OF THE GOAT

"I WONDER WHAT'S IN STORE FOR US THIS YEAR"

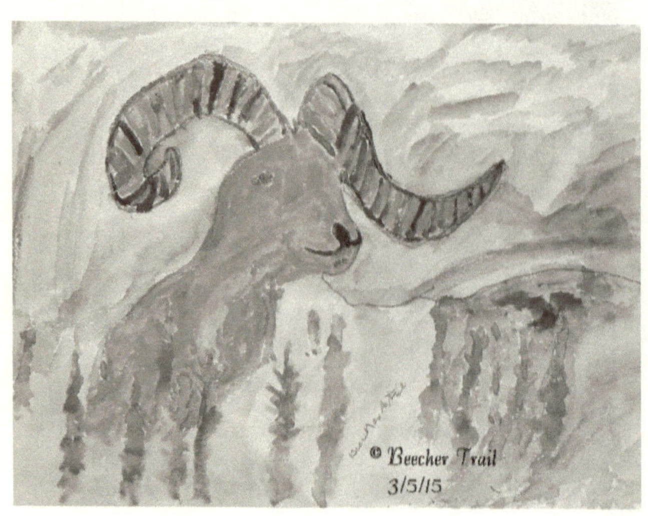

"Big Horn Sheep"
Watercolor by Beecher Trail
"Goats help take care of your emotional, spiritual and mental well-being and help you get rid of guilty feelings"

January 4

Beecher took razor blades in his fanny pack to Day Care and tried shaving and cut his face up pretty good because they were dull. Poor guy! It didn't even seem to bother him.

~

January 12

I took Beecher to his appointment at the VA. Beecher still sees all the doctors at the VA as well as Dr. Léger at the Brain Center. They agreed to co-manage since Beecher needs all the doctors involved in his care. Today he had his TB Test and his pneumonia and flu shot. He needs the TB test yearly to be able to go to Day Care. His primary doctor's nurse asked when was the last time Beecher had a colonoscopy and I said I wasn't sure. She recommended he have one, but in the meantime, she sent him home with a stool sample test to be returned within 48 hours. She told me to follow up with a colonoscopy. I am not sure about this and will address it with Dr. Léger.

~

January 8

Beecher fell at Adult Day Care. Stood up, started shaking and fell over backwards. An aide tried to break his fall, but he fell on her. She didn't get hurt, thank God! Blood pressure was 135/105. Wouldn't eat lunch but I told nurse to make him eat. He finally did and his blood pressure went down to 135/85.

He lost his wallet and iPhone at day care again.

He opened a jar of honey that I just had bought and got his cup ready for coffee for the next day. He spilled honey all over the floor; about ¼ cup. Didn't even know he did it.

~

January 11

This morning he spilled dairy creamer all over the floor and some in the recycle bin. My mop sure is getting a lot of use, and my nerves are about shot. Beecher told me he found his wallet but couldn't tell me where he found it. Just keeps repeating that it is in his pants.

~

January 19

I still haven't found his iPhone. He now says a guy named Jesse in a wheelchair at Day Care has it. He repeatedly says it and won't answer how he knows. Says Jesse stole it from him. Called the day care and they said there is no one there named Jesse. Hallucination or had a dream? I just don't know anymore.

I ran into an old friend at a book signing. One of our friend's daughters has a lot of the same symptoms as Beech. She is 54, has aphasia, gorges her food, has had a lot of car accidents and a blank stare on her face. I encouraged her to go to the Lou Ruvo Brain Center for a diagnosis as it seems to me it could be FTD.

We are missing arm covers for the chair we have on loan from NAN (Neighbors Assisting Neighbors, a community service to help seniors since we live in a community of over 55 residents). Beecher is using a remote hydraulic chair which lifts him almost to a standing position. All of a sudden, the covers are missing. He doesn't know what happened to them.

Everything seems to be moving faster these days, more dropping things, bigger messes in the kitchen, clothes everywhere in bathroom, continues to shave with a razor he took out of the trash. I told him several days ago to start using his electric shaver. He has no social skills, no phone etiquette, and unacceptable behavior in public. When he eats and drops something on the floor, he picks it up and puts it in his mouth.

Continues to do everything I tell him not to, i.e. no ice cream or shakes in the morning; won't finish his meals while he's sitting down; walks to the kitchen with a fork or spoon full of food, dropping it as he goes. He ignores me when I tell him not to. Most of the time, I can't understand him. Out of the blue, he talks about things that I have no idea what he's talking about. This is getting harder and harder all the time. FTD is never the same. It ebbs and flows like a river that is taking away our loved one as far as it can, never to return to the norm. We keep hoping the river will return them to us the way they were before as we hopelessly try to save them. As he continues to disappear right before my eyes, I feel myself disappearing too and I pray that later when this ordeal is over that I will find myself again. I sometimes feel jealous of other people that I see that are happy and carefree, the couples with their arms around each other, they seem so out of place in my world and yet I long for that feeling of utopia again.

Tomorrow, he has an appointment with the Orthopedic doctor to get measured for compression socks. Sometime in the next few months, he will start physical therapy to determine what kind of walker he should have. No falls in the last two weeks. Thank goodness!

~

January 20

Beecher got his compression socks today. After we got home, I was going over the instructions about how to put them on. I asked him what was the first thing he was supposed to do after he got out of the shower. He said, "Make sure my feet are wrinkle free!" I laughed so hard and he thought it was so funny too. I told him, "No, the girl said you're supposed to make sure your feet are completely dry before you put the socks on." I guess he remembered the girl at the orthopedic place told him to make sure he got his socks all the way up, and make sure there are no wrinkles (in the socks). So funny! So nice to get a laugh from him and I haven't laughed that hard in a long time!

January 21

After dinner tonight as I was getting ready for bed, he walked in the bathroom and said as clear as a bell, and he was looking directly at me, "Take a rest for a while."

January 22

Another day of frustration. Beecher got out my gel pens just as I was trying to get lunch on the table. He dropped the whole carousel and all the pens fell out. Later that day he pulled the lamp over to him that was on the other side of my chair so he could turn the light on. It hit him on the head and knocked off the top lamp piece.

January 25

I took him to see the movie American Sniper. He cried hard at the end. There is still a little empathy left in him.

January 26

Beecher fell getting out of the recliner by tripping over the blanket.

Need to solve this problem but don't know how. Frances the nanny helped me rearrange the living room to prevent falls. Took us about two hours!

January 27

Typical day. Beecher ate a good dinner and all of it for a change. Beecher came into the kitchen and got the funnel out of the drawer. I asked him what he needed it for. He said he didn't know.

~

January 28

Beecher got up and had the strainer out. Asked him what for and he said "To strain the milk." He had milk with his cookies last night and poured the leftover milk back in the carton so he strained it to use in his coffee. He didn't know I had more milk in the outside fridge.

I sent a message to Dr Léger as follows: I need your advice on something. At Beecher's last visit to his primary doctor at the VA, the nurse asked when was the last time he had a colonoscopy. Being that it's been over 10 years, she said he should have one. Do you think it's medically necessary? Being his primary doctor, I know she doesn't understand or know much about FTD. I don't think he could get through the prep, let alone get thru the night, and then keep him from having food or water until the test. His progression of the disease seems to be speeding up, falling and losing his balance a lot. They said he has a lot of Parkinson symptoms and his attention span is terrible. Most of the time he will not answer me when I talk to him. They issued compression stockings and may want to give him a walker after he does some physical therapy. He's much worse in many areas and he is definitely a handful. I respect your opinion so please give me your thoughts. This is Dr Léger's response.

It's a difficult call. We don't want any patient to not undergo standard of care treatments or investigations just because they have a neurodegenerative condition, but you are right about how difficult the preparation, let alone the actual procedure will be for him, and with what benefit? Maybe you could discuss with them alternatives such as serial occult blood or even CT colonoscopy, which may require less preparation. None-the-less, unless there is a very strong history of colon cancer in the family, it may be better to be more conservative at this point. I'm sorry if this seems a little ambivalent, although nuanced may be a better choice or word. Try as much as possible to keep him active, but take care of yourself.

That assured me that it was unnecessary and I reported that back to his primary doctor.

〜

January 29

Watercolor day is every Thursday. Don't know if it de-stresses me or not anymore. Beecher knocked over his chair twice, doesn't follow instructions, makes messes and is always getting into my supplies and he has all his own supplies. I think he enjoys it more because most of the time I am cleaning up after him.

We ran some errands after class and then stopped at Taco Bell. After he finished eating, he went to the bathroom. On the way he took his cup of soda to refill but left it on a counter on the way. I was afraid someone would throw it away so I put it back on our table. As he was coming back, I saw that he had picked up someone else's cup. I told him I had his cup and he proceeded to set it down on the edge of the counter and it spilled. I immediately jumped up and saw that it belonged to a little boy and I went to the counter to ask the clerk if the boy could have another cup and to clean up the spill. Went back to our table to clean up our table and grabbed my phone. Beecher was already walking out. I looked around for the boy and saw the sister refilling the cup. As I walked out the door, I saw a lady yelling at someone and I saw that it was Beecher. He was by our car and he started walking towards her. I told him to go back to the car. She was the mother of the kids. I apologized and tried to explain about Beecher's condition. She just kept saying he should have apologized. I tried again to explain his condition and then she said, "He looks fine to me," with an attitude no less. She turned to get in her car and I motioned the little boy to roll down his window. I apologized and explained to him that my husband has a problem with his brain and he didn't mean to take his drink. I think he understood more than the mother! With tears in my eyes at this point I looked at the mother and said, "I have to deal with this every day. At least you should have some compassion." I walked away.

I'm learning that I have to be an advocate and protect him as if he were a child. It's heartbreaking. With FTD you are constantly apologizing for behavior and you're constantly grieving the loss of someone you haven't lost yet. My child, my husband; no one really understands. It is so sad. I no longer know what "normal" is; I only know that it isn't. When I think back on these last few years and everything that has happened, I can only relate to anyone who is going through the same experience and the loss I feel is overwhelming. His sister Ruth once said the disease transformed him into someone he wouldn't want to be. He was aware of everything but locked up in his body as it deteriorated around him. That is so true. I guess it's a good thing he's not even aware of it.

$\sim$

January 30

Thank goodness today is day care! While waiting for transportation to pick him up, he said his girlfriend is going to be there today. I asked him who his girlfriend was and he said Suzanne. She hasn't been there for two weeks. I said is that why he always had to dress sharp and he said yes. I don't know how I feel about this. Don't think its jealousy. Just think I feel hurt and don't know how to explain it.

Today I got approved for another grant from the Alzheimer's Organization, which is good for seven more weeks starting Jan. 30-March 30. I know I'm going to need it!

Well, I thought I would get some rest. Day Care brought him home an hour and a half early. Didn't call or anything. Good thing I was home. That shortened my alone time. Also, they picked him up late this morning which has become their routine lately. Spent part of the day trying to figure out the invoice from ADC. Says I owe them money. I should be even with them. I try not to do any business on my one day alone. But it never fails. When do I get some time for myself? I know, I'm whining again!

⌇

February 4

Another upsetting day. Started out good other than this cough I have. Felt good enough to go to the movies and lunch with the girls from dance. We saw "Black or White" with Kevin Costner. Excellent movie!

Frances was here to watch Beecher. Came home and took a nap and woke up feeling yucky. Fixed dinner for Beecher. Told him I was going to Walgreens to get some meds for my cough. Told him I would clean up the pans when I got back and to not touch anything.

When I got back, I saw that my George Foreman grill was broken. He had cleaned it and dropped it. Thank goodness he didn't get hurt. But I was mad he broke it after I told him to leave things alone. I can't even count how many dishes he has broken the last two years!

⌇

February 5

He seems to be having trouble with telling time. I had him draw a clock and put in the numbers. The numbers were off a bit but he got all of them and in order.

At 10 am he was turning down the covers for bed and had his backpack packed for tomorrow's day care. He had already packed it the night before. He seems to be getting more confused with the time of day. Another upset! He deleted some of my TV shows again! Probably the tenth time in the last year!

⌇

February 6

Today is my mother's birthday. She would have been 91 today. My friend Susan took me out and treated me to a pedicure and lunch. That was very thoughtful of her. Beecher was at Day Care so it was a relaxing day. Since he got home, he's been speaking very softly. I can hardly hear him.

~

February 7

He's getting worse. Every day is a new challenge. He never listens to my commands. We had to go to our grandson's house to look at a chair. Ran some errands while we were out. Doesn't seem to understand the word "stop" or "wait.' Doesn't seem to know what opposite means. Everything is such a chore for him. He continues to stand up to take his jeans off while he constantly wobbles and almost falls down. He sometimes sits on the chair in the closet and even falls off of it. Came home from the store and he started pouring his drink into another cup while standing two feet away from the sink instead of over the sink. He spilled it all over the floor that Frances had just mopped before she went home. It's so tiring day after day.

~

February 8

One of his new habits is unscrewing the lid on his Sippy cup while he's sitting in the recliner (quite some time ago I bought him a child's Sippy Cup because he spills so much and the cup has a lid on it and cuts down the amount of spillage, if you know what I mean) By the time he gets to the kitchen he usually has it spilled. Tonight, he spilled almost a full glass and didn't even know it. Just left it and refilled his cup and walked back to his chair while screwing the lid on.

He told me tonight his friend Kim doesn't like him anymore. He won't return his calls. Feel so sorry for him. None of his friends keep in touch. So sad. I think he calls him too much and Kim doesn't know what to say to him. It's so hard to communicate with him.

~

February 10

I got up this morning to find the freezer door half open. Everything thawed out. I think I will go look for refrigerator locks so he can't get into the fridge. He must have left it open when he got ice for his water glass last night. This just happens way too often. I can't keep up with him. Hard as I try, I can't follow him from room to room all day long.

~

February 13 (Friday the 13th)

I went to quick care. I have pneumonia. I have to stay low and rest to get better. Thank goodness I have Frances coming tomorrow. I have to get well so I can keep taking care of The Beech!

~

February 14

Valentine's Day! No going out to dinner until I get well. Frances bought a Valentine card and helped Beecher sign it and he gave it to me along with a bottle of wine she bought me. That was so thoughtful of her. Had an interesting night. Beecher ate a special pot cookie someone had given him and got super wasted. Started getting up and down repeatedly in his chair. Got up to go to bed and could hardly get his pants off. Broke his belt. Came out of room with his underwear half on and holding his pjs. Went into closet and tried to get him to pull up his underwear. Finally told him to sit on the floor and I tried to get him to pull up his underwear but he couldn't do it sitting down. He seemed so weak and unable to move. Kept trying to get him to stand up by pulling himself up on the doorjamb. He had a hard time doing that. I finally helped pull him up. He was so disoriented. Took him to bed and he said in a baby voice, "You're treating me like a baby." He was laughing and liking it. He finally went to sleep and slept eleven hours. Maybe I should give him more cookies but it may not be so safe; still, he was happy for a while.

February 15

Well today he took apple seeds out to the backyard two different times and said he planted a majestic apple tree. Wonder where they came from. Maybe because I told him we had to stop feeding the birds. Frances usually cuts up and puts out the core of the apples for them.

February 16

The day started off with Beecher waking up at 5 am and taking a shower. He did however close the door to the bathroom while he showered. But then left the bedroom door open. Went into living room and turned the TV on high and both lights in the kitchen on.

So, I didn't get back to sleep. Then he fixed himself some cream of wheat and spilled a whole glass of milk on the floor and brown sugar all over the stove top.

Doesn't seem fair. He should be taking care of me instead of me taking care of him. I need to rest as much as possible.

I know I'm having a pity party! But this is the toughest thing I've ever dealt with in my life.

February 17

He's going to Day Care today so I'll get some rest! Today was as usual. What is usual, is not what used to be normal. He told me he couldn't find his wallet. I was sure he had it when he came home from day care on Friday. Seems all I do most days is look for the remotes to the TV or other objects he carries from room to room. Such as, his chair pillow, reading glasses and sunglasses. Blue gremlins (toothpicks) are dropped everywhere all over the house. And now I'm finding Q-tips in odd places. It's a challenge every day.

His obsessive behaviors are a different story. He always makes sure he has his backpack ready for day care including toothbrush with tooth-paste on it, some candy and enough toothpicks and baby wipes to last three days! He doesn't ask for them much anymore when he's at home, only when he goes to Day Care. I have to check his backpack several times to make sure he doesn't have anything in there that he shouldn't (like a razor blade)! Tonight, I found five sleeping aid pills in with his Tums. He went through my bathroom drawers and found them. He thought they were Aleve. Good thing I checked. He would have been passed out at day care all day or worse.

I try to keep one step ahead of him but I never know what he's going to do next. I hide as much as possible from him including his meds which I dole out to him twice a day. I'm running out of places to hide things.

After dinner I had to set up a new remote for the TV. He can't do that stuff anymore. Everything is left to me to fix. Anyway, I took the wrapper off the remote as he was walking into the kitchen to get a drink. He had his Sippy cup in his hand and I asked him to come get the wrapper and throw it away for me. He walked toward me with the top off the cup and spilled what was left in the cup and all the ice. About eight cubes.

Took him a couple of minutes to pick them up. Kept trying to hold them all in one hand rather than put them back in cup. Pick two up. Drop one.

He really is getting worse. Seems more like a two-year-old now instead of a five-year-old. I hate what is happening to him and can't do anything about it. I'm so frustrated all the time. Went to bed at 9. Before he went to sleep, he said he left a book at day care that they gave him. He said it was about wee care. I told him I would call and have them save it for him. And then he said, "I'm sorry I'm such a big pain in the ass." His first words of empathy in a long time. I cried so hard for both of us. I hugged him and held him and assured him I would not leave him. I told him how much I loved him and that we would get through this together. Told him I wished I could do something to change what was happening to him. He told me he loved me and went to sleep. I continued to cry to let out some held in emotions. Got a good night's sleep. Crying helped.

February 18

Ok day. I'm feeling better. Frances was here today. I got some much-needed rest. Beech always leaves his blanket on the floor in front of his chair and almost trips on it every time he gets up. I remind him constantly but it does no good. So today Frances and I figured out if I put the soft stool next to his chair and told him if he put it there every time he got up for one full day, she would bring him a coconut cupcake next time she comes. She made him practice a few times. He seems to be doing good so far.

February 20

Every day is different. Found an empty yogurt container in the bathroom along with a spoon. Not the first time. I've found candy wrappers too. Guess he sits on the toilet and eats.

February 22

I took a video of him reading his daily affirmation from his NA book. He can still read a lot of the words but much slower and quieter. Slurs most of the small words. He didn't know I was taping him on my iPhone. When he finished, he looked up at me and I told him I was taping him. I asked him if he wanted to say something to me and he smiled and said "Love you." I said "I love you too and that he had read very good." My eyes teared up. It was a very special moment to have him look at me that way while saying those words.

He is also having problems with the remote. Turns it off a lot when he means to hit another button. When I ask him what he wants for lunch, he doesn't answer me. Asked him five or six times. No response. He does this a lot. Finally asked him if he wanted a grilled cheese and he said yes. Amy is taking him to the movies this afternoon.

After the movies, Amy bought dinner at Raising Canes. Yummy! He didn't eat much. He always orders more and saves for lunch the next day. He spent a lot of time on his iPad when he got home. He makes me so nervous. He almost fell three times while standing up and playing his iPad. He almost sat on the end table once and the next time he landed on the arm of the chair and fell into the chair. He doesn't pay attention to what he is doing. The blanket is still a problem too.

February 23

Rough day! I took him to the VA for appt. for his meds. He sat in the chair waiting to see the doctor while playing his iPad and constantly leaning into me. He was not even aware. Visit went well. Drove home and made several stops for groceries; Sam's Club, Walmart, 99cent store and Vons. I needed some things from each store. When we were in Walmart, I let him get some ice cream. When we got to the check stand and I had everything on the counter, he walked away heading back to the groceries. I asked him three times where he was going. He didn't answer me. He just kept on walking. I figured he went to get something he wanted. As the checker was finishing up with the customer in front of me, I looked around to see where he was. I saw him two aisles over standing in front of another checker. I saw she had rung up something and put it in a bag and he was starting to walk away. I excused myself from the line and told my checker I had to take care of my husband at another lane. When I got to where he was, the checker said he hadn't paid for the food and she took some Hershey's chocolate out of the bag and asked if I wanted it. I apologized and told her no. I was at another check stand. I went back and paid for my stuff and left. Told him he couldn't do that anymore. He does not carry any money on him. He just doesn't understand. He only knows what he wants. Glad the checker was ok with the situation. She could have accused him of stealing. He was being very stubborn when I handed the chocolate back to the checker. Guess I'm not going to take him to the store anymore. I ended up stopping at another store to get the Hershey's chocolate for him.

I'm not done writing yet. Really rough day! I called him to the table for dinner. It took me getting up and calling him five times. He was playing with his iPad. He ate a pretty good dinner. After he finished, he went over to pick up his iPad again. I was still eating. All of a sudden, I heard him fall. He was on the floor and the recliner chair was knocked backwards. I was only three feet away. I did not see it happen. He said he was alright. I tried to find out what happened. He didn't answer. My guess is he was playing his game on the iPad and went to sit in the chair and didn't pay attention to where he was sitting and missed the chair or just fell back into it causing it to go backwards. He's a big guy. 6'2" and weighs 245. After I helped him up, he grabbed his iPad and walked over to his other chair that he normally sits in and before I could stop him, he was already falling into that chair sideways. It didn't even faze him. At least he didn't knock it over. This is not fun! He's getting worse and I can't watch him every second. Where and when will this all end? I do not know. It scares me. That's enough for today. I hope.

~

February 25

My Father died on this day 45 years ago today. I had a day to myself. Beech was at Day Care all day. I so enjoy my time alone. One day a week is not enough. I had a lot of calls to make to set him up for the new day care he starts next week. I just sat down to relax for the last hour before he was due home. (I really enjoy that last hour.) I didn't get it.

Transportation brought him home early at 4:20 instead of 5:30. This is the third time they brought him home that early. I was very upset and told the driver I told the person in charge last week they were bringing him too early. She said she would fix it but she didn't. It's a shame I don't look forward to him coming home but I value every minute he's gone. Plus, I could have been gone when they dropped him off. He has no key to get in so he would have been left alone outside, or taken back to Day Care, or I would have left my errand to come back home. Guess I will call again to let them know I'm upset. This is supposed to be respite time for me.

$\sim$

February 28

A typical day. A lot of telling him to pick up his blanket so he won't trip over it. He just ignores me. I don't know why I bother. He's not going to get better. He's just getting worse. He played Scrabble with Frances today. He does fairly well.

While watching TV, he told me his girlfriend, Suzanne wasn't at day care on Friday. Guess he missed saying goodbye to her. It was his last day at that Day Care. Today he put his t-shirt on backwards. He wasn't even aware of it. Sometimes he puts it on inside out.

Next week he starts at the new Day Care in Henderson. Only problem is they can't pick him up from our home. I had to find a place of business which is about three miles from where we live and the bus will come there and pick him up and return him there at the end of the day, and then I have to go there to pick him up.

~

March 2

What a day! He's so incoherent most of the time. He does not listen to me. He does not answer me. Took me ten minutes to figure out what he wanted for dinner. I think I am going to quit asking him what he wants for dinner and just give him two choices. He kept changing his mind. Over and over, I repeated back to him. And still could not get a straight answer from him. After dinner he was up and down at least twenty times! Three times was to fill his water cup. He kept adding new ice and water three times within fifteen minutes. He constantly kept tripping over his blanket and losing the TV remote control every five minutes. I finally took it away from him because I got tired of looking for it. One of the new things he has starting doing is emptying the kitchen trash when it is only half full. He doesn't understand that he is wasting the bags. Also, he sits at the table as soon as I start preparing meals or dessert. I always tell him it won't be ready for a while. In the last ten minutes he got up three times again to fill his water glass and he hasn't even drunk much. This repetition is driving me crazy!!

Another thing he does is constantly change the TV station. He will watch a show for fifteen or twenty minutes and then switch to another station. Usually something he had recorded. Ten minutes later he will switch again. This happens daily over and over.

I found out today that I can get five days of respite care. I've applied for a grant to go to an AFTD seminar in San Diego in April. My daughters are going with me. In order to get Beecher in a nursing home for five days while I'm gone, I had to submit an "Inpatient Respite Consultation and be referred by his primary doctor. He will also have to have a chest x-ray. I contacted a social worker at the VA to start the process. It is best to do one to two weeks in advance or even sooner as to guarantee I can get him in the home when I need it. The minimum stay is five days (which is perfect as the seminar is two days, and my daughters and I plan to stay an extra day and then still have two days left to myself when I get home). The social worker sent me some names of the nursing homes to check out. Keeping my fingers crossed! If this works out, I can apply up to 30 days per year! I don't even have to be gone anywhere. I can just stay home and have five days to myself six times a year. Yes, this would be a blessing!

~

March 3

Just when I think I've had the roughest day ever; I get surprised with a worse one. The day started with Beecher waking me up at 5:30. Took his shower and then left bedroom door open. I couldn't get back to sleep. A half hour later, he kept going out to the backyard and looking around. He ate an apple and then went to the garage to get a tool to dig a hole to plant an apple seed.

I took him with me to my doctor appointment. As I went in to see the nurse, Beecher went to the bathroom. Doctor came in and then he went to the bathroom again. As I was talking to the doc in the office area he walked over and picked up one of the employee's water bottles. He had brought a bottle in with him and I guess he thought it was his.

Made a few stops on the way home and then to Taco Bell. He got two burritos. Ate one and then went to the counter to get a lid for the green sauce and a bag for the other burrito he hadn't eaten. He then walked straight to the men's room with the bag. He came out about ten minutes later. Only thing left in the bag was the green sauce. He said he ate some of the burrito and threw the rest in the toilet or trash. It was time to go!

After we got home and I noticed he had two bottles of soda open. He had his plastic Sippy cup in the fridge with ice cream already in it. He went to get one of the sodas but I told him no. Told him to use the soda he brought home from Taco Bell. He did. But he spilled most of it on the floor and counter. Mopped that up and told him he couldn't have any more soda the rest of the day. Water only I told him.

Fifteen minutes later, as I was just sitting down to relax, I heard him in the kitchen opening a bottle of soda. By the time I got to the kitchen, he had most of it sprayed all over both sinks, half of the kitchen floor, down the door of the dishwasher and most of the counter space on two parts of the counters. I just about lost it!! He just stood there like a two-year-old not even aware of what he had done or remember that I told him, no more soda. And the day is only half over!!!

One of the things I miss is going out with him on a date and I look at other couples and think how fortunate they are to be spending a regular night out. It's such a drastic reminder of how far from reality I am. Wishful thinking never got you anywhere. Some days I don't even recognize myself. I feel like I'm on another planet or in a nightmare. I don't feel like a participant in any aspect of my life. I'm just an observer as I watch him disappear more and more each day. I often think about everything I've ever taken for granted and realize I forgot to stop and smell the roses. I miss those roses, the ones he gave me every Valentines, Anniversaries and my birthday without fail. Not a year would go by, that I didn't get the roses. He was such a romantic and now he doesn't even know what day it is. I was recently reminded to not wait for things to get easier, simpler, or better because life will always be complicated. Learn to be happy right now; otherwise, you'll run out of time. Well, I don't know how to be happy right now--it's too complicated. Guess I'd better go smell some roses.

March 4

I got approval for new Adult Day Care in Henderson. He will be going every Friday starting next week. I talked to them about a grant that they have, that will let him go two to three times a week and won't cost me anything. Told them I would start with once a week until he gets used to the new place. This will be such a relief as I really need some down time.

Frances will still be coming several times a week, including Saturday if I need her, or she will come in the evening when I do to my Support Group meeting at the Brain Center.

March 5

Constant spills in kitchen. Not much else to report. We went to watercolor. He painted a picture for Dr. Léger of a big horn sheep. He's going to give it to him tomorrow when he goes for his sixth month follow up.

Kept hearing a rattle in my car and decided it might be my donut tire not tightened down. Frances was over and we tried to figure out how to do it. The car manual wasn't much help. I finally asked Beech to help us since he used to bust tires down in his dad's tire shop. That wasn't a good idea! First of all, he didn't listen to what I was telling him that we were trying to do. He kept taking the tire to side of car like he was going to change the tire. Then he kept trying to put the tire back in car. I wanted him to show me how to tighten the jack in the trunk. He almost tripped over the mat cover. He just didn't get it. I finally told him to go back in the house. A man walking with his wife stopped to help us. I'm happy to say, the rattle had stopped! Yay!

~

March 6

We went to visit to Dr Léger today. He said Beech is pretty healthy. Weight and blood pressure good. He wants to do blood work for genetic testing in a few weeks. Also wants him off of Seroquel and wants to put him on Lexapro. He said he feels Beech is about half way (about midway in the moderate stage) in the disease. He added in notes that he now has Corticobasal Syndrome. He says there is no harm in his playing his iPad. Also, he has Parkinsonism not Parkinson's disease. I told him of having problems tying shoes and picking up things like ice cubes. And also, about the repetitive actions (refilling his mug every few minutes) and also repeating things to me over and over. He told me to watch for swallowing problems.

I also told him of all the falls he's had. Told him VA is doing physical therapy to determine if and when he needs a walker. Dr Léger said there could be more problems with it. So, we'll see. Beech gave him the picture he painted. He said he was not used to accepting gifts but he would and he liked it very much!

Exam today showed his gait was slightly stooped, he showed no arm swing and had increased urinary frequency. He generally goes to the bathroom several times when we are there. He noted that Beech had undergone the swallowing assessment at the VA and it was felt to be normal. In addition to the other assessment of diagnosis, he has now added Parkinsonism with features of both CBD (Corticobasal Dementia) and PSP (Progressive Supranuclear Palsy). Progressive Supranuclear Palsy is another type of FTD disorder and shares some of the same symptoms with bvFTD. i.e., gait and balance disturbance, generally falling backwards, visual disturbance with the inability to coordinate eye movements, inability to look up or down and sometimes unable to keep their eyes open. The progression of PSP is more rapid than bvFTD. Dr. Léger changed his medication. He is now on Escitalopram Oxalate.

~

March 7

This will be a month to remember. Beecher sat down for lunch at home. I asked him if he had a glass of soda anywhere. He said no he didn't want any. A minute later he started to get up and fell backwards falling off the chair and hitting the ground. He tried to get up but couldn't. I had to help him. I asked if he was hurt and he said no. Then finally he said he hit the back of his head. I checked but no bump. He always gets up several times while he's eating for some reason or other. I thought I heard a crack when he fell. I checked the chair and it was cracked. Another thing broken, but at least he's not hurt. He is destroying so many things. How will I ever get through this?

I told him I would take him to Red Lobster tonight. We still have a gift card my brother Donny gave us for Christmas. After Beecher finished eating lunch, he went in and started getting ready for dinner. I stopped him and told him it was only 12:30. He got his t-shirt and slippers back on. Ten minutes later he had changed into dress clothes. Oh well!

We had a nice dinner. He ate well and no spills or too big of a mess. After we got home, we watched Glee and a movie I rented. He was up and down about ten times refilling his water glass. Also, he couldn't turn on the chair remote. He tried ten times before he got it turned on. He kept moving chair back and forth. Constantly!! This is driving me crazy!!! Finally turned off TV and went to bed.

Another day tomorrow to face! What will it be like I wonder? Well, I thought the day was over. Not!! He just spilled a whole glass of water and ice cubes next to his side of the bed. Don't know why he had the lid unscrewed.

~

March 8

Uneventful day except for stuff spilled everywhere. I probably mopped kitchen floor at least five times. He still can't figure out the chair remote. I've showed him at least twenty times in the last two days. He just doesn't understand. It's so tiring.

~

March 10

Went to watercolor by myself. First time in weeks. Felt so good to get out and do something I enjoy so much. Frances was here to watch Beecher.

Another day of trying to communicate with him. He kept changing his drink cups. Filling one up then pouring it out. Just after he poured a whole glass of root beer, he started to pour it out. I figured out why. He was ready for his milkshake. I stopped him and made him drink the rest of it. After the milkshake, he filled his glass with water. He carried it into the bedroom. The lid was missing. Looked for it for over a half hour. An hour later it appeared on his glass!! I asked him where he found it. He said under the end table. I know I looked there. It amazes me how many times a day he loses things.

~

March 11

We went to lunch with his friends Keith and Kim. Beech was on good behavior. No spills or getting up and down. I had a nice time and I think Beecher was glad to see his friends. It's sad because even when I'm out with him and friends, I feel like a part of me is missing. I no longer feel like his wife, but just his caregiver. I have to do all the talking as he can't relate to his friends. I sure would like the normal back in my life but it doesn't appear to be found anywhere. I'm becoming a whiner and nobody likes a whiner but I just can't help it. I need normalcy in my life.

Took him to 99 cent store and he bought some probiotic drinks. Didn't know they were frozen. He let them thaw out and drank five at a time. He spilled most of them on the floor, counter and inside the fridge. What a mess!

~

March 12

Beecher's first visit to the Nevada Adult Day Care in Henderson started.

I had transferred him there because there was more opportunity to get a state grant. The only problem was they could not pick him up from the house and the RTC buses on that run did not come to our neighborhood. I found a small restaurant about eight minutes away where they could pick him up. I had to call the night before to find out the approximate pickup time and the return time within five minutes and make sure I had him there in time. I had to wait in the car until they picked him up and be there when they dropped him off. I had instructed Beecher to wait inside the restaurant in case for any reason he was dropped off early or I was late. I had informed the management that he might occasionally be coming inside. I explained our situation and his disease so they didn't think he was a homeless person. He came home from day care with a different pair of pants on. He had a bag with his soiled pants and underwear in it. He said he wet himself. I told him to put them in the wash and Frances would wash on Saturday. I called the Day Care. They said he spilled juice on them but it smelled like urine to me. They keep extra clothes for accidents.

~

March 13

Day Care Day again. Yay! I decided to let him go 2 days a week. It gives me more respite time. I picked him up from the bus stop and took him to dinner at Taco Y Taco. He finished eating way before me. He kept getting up from table to refill his soda cup. The third time he spilled the whole large cup all over the floor, table and chair. I apologized to the family eating next to us. I can't even take him to a fast-food place without him making a mess. One of the things about his illness is that I can never expect the days to be the same. He will hardly ever turn off the light in the bathroom. I have to remind him all the time. But every time I am in the bathroom doing my hair or getting ready or in the shower, he will walk in and brush his teeth and turn off the light after he's done. Never fails!

~

March 14

I took him to the VA for physical therapy. PT said he was 18 out of 24 on the risk scale; 18 being low risk, but felt he could use some therapy. We stopped at In -N-Out for lunch on the way home. Mistake! Made a mess and then walked out to car before I finished. Didn't know where he was.

It scares me when he does that. When am I going to learn? Expect the unexpected all the time. He really is like a two-year-old.

~

March 16

It was a nice and easy day for a change. Beech was at Day Care all day. I went to Walmart and bought some locks for the fridge to keep him out, but they didn't fit our fridge. I try to keep a lot of things in the freezer and fridge in the garage since he usually doesn't go out there. I also bought some motion detector plug in lights for the bathroom so he can see if he gets up in the middle of the night. Less chance he will fall. He made me a St. Patrick's card with four leaf clovers at Day Care. Picked him up from bus stop and came home and ate dinner. Other than making a mess when he made his milkshake, he wasn't too bad. He was in a quiet mood. He wanted to know when he goes back to Day Care. I think he likes it there. Got a call from the social worker at the VA and they have ordered Beecher's chest-x-ray. He can go in anytime as a walk in.

~

March 18

Day care again today! Beecher got up in a quiet mood. Ate two yogurts and an apple. Stuffed some sweet tarts in his pocket. I took them out and reminded him he can't take candy to day care. (He might give some to someone that has diabetes). Noticed that he didn't put any baby wipes in his man bag. Didn't say anything to him. He made the bed today. He usually makes it every day except the days he goes to day care.

Going to lunch with my daughter Amy today! What a day! Started out as I decided to go back to dance class after being off since I was sick with pneumonia. Turned my ankle and got a bad sprain; only hurt when I first did it. Came home and iced it. Felt better so Amy picked me up for lunch. Was ok to walk until I got home three hours later when it started hurting. Iced it again for two hours. Then picked Beecher up from the bus and drove to quick care up the street. Three hours there with x-rays, getting a splint on and of course learning how- to- walk- in crutches. Made it to the pharmacy just in time to get scripts. In a splint and crutches now. Home at 10 pm. Heated up leftover cabbage rolls for us. That was fun!! NOT! Trying to get around the kitchen on crutches while trying to get Beecher to help me. He was so out of it, he couldn't understand my commands. Was so frustrating for me! Then he spilled some condensed milk on floor. What a mess. Will have to get Frances to mop the floor again. Thank God she is coming over tomorrow. Finally got to bed at 11 pm. Ice pack on foot every 20 minutes and propped up foot on pillow with no one to help me. He is just not capable. He makes everything harder for me instead of helping me. That's just the way it is these days. Hope I heal soon. Have to see a specialist ASAP. Also need to get him to bus stop tomorrow for Day Care. Hard to drive with this splint on and not safe either. At least I'll have the day to myself! Will have to get someone to drive me to specialist. This is such a drag!! Can't get appt until April 2. Hope I'll be well be then!

As I was going to bed, I noticed the top of my Lortabs bottle that the doctor prescribed was not screwed on right. I counted my pills and one was missing. I asked Beech if he got into my pills. He said no and then a few minutes later he walked out of the bedroom with one in his hand. Asked him where he got it and he pointed to the bedroom. I immediately hid the bottle of pills. I should have known better!

March 20

Went to bed at 9:30. Woke up at 11:30. My foot was screaming! Got up and went into the guest room. Took the splint off. I think the ace wrap was too tight. Once I took it off it felt better. Left it off, propped up my foot and fell right back to sleep. Slept until 4:20. Back to sleep and alarm woke me at 5. Slept like a baby. Needed it. I think the pills helped!

Videotaped Beech tying his shoes. Took him over three minutes and still didn't get one tied. I had to do it for him. The last few days he has seemed much more confused and hardly talking at all and when he does it's a whisper. Every task seems complicated and confusing. I think it's time I get serious about what I need to do.

Since he got home from Day Care, he has been very unsteady. Bumped into stool and then into chair and fell on his butt. Didn't get hurt. Almost fell again in kitchen. Seems like he's drugged. He's talking in whispers if he talks at all.

My next-door neighbor took me to Redbox to drop off movie. Beech wanted to go with us. When we got home, he almost fell again getting out of the car. He had taken his shoes off in the car before he got out of the car.

～

March 23

Another day of losing his balance. He was standing up and playing his iPad and leaning into it. Almost fell sideways. Then when Frances was here, he ran into the chair and almost fell. He doesn't pay attention to where he's going. He spent most of the day on his iPad sitting in the same position for hours and hours.

Today I noted changes in his eating habits. He takes his time lifting his utensils to his mouth, very slowly. Prior to this he shoveled his food into his mouth.

～

March 25

My sister Linda was visiting, so my sisters, Linda and Patti and I drove to Mt. Charleston to have lunch. It was a nice day, and good to get out of the house. When we got home, my daughters were at the house when Beecher fell out of the kitchen chair. He got out of the chair and started falling backwards. He almost fell into the wall where a big mirror hung.

Michelle banged her knee on the chair, and Linda was able to brace his fall. It scared all of us but he didn't get hurt.

~

March 27

I found out today from the VA that I got confirmed for the five-day Respite Care. He will stay in the facility I choose while I go to the Conference in San Diego with my daughters next month. It took some time to get him confirmed. He will be staying at Silver Hills Health Care Center. It is a locked facility, lots of activities, two people to a room, TV in room. I will have to mark all his clothes with his initials and send a copy of his Health Power of Attorney, copy of directive, and list of meds. Yay!!!

~

April 2

I've had bad allergies for days. I haven't written in this journal in several days. I'll try to catch up. This is the way our day went. Frances isn't coming until tonight so I can go to a watercolor reception. I asked Beecher if he wanted to go to watercolor class. He said no. So, I decided to leave him home alone for a few hours since I was only a few blocks away. Mistake #1 for the day! I told him to eat a tuna sandwich which I had made or some pasta I made last night. He can heat up in the microwave.

I came home and the back door was wide open. I saw a pan on stove so I knew he had cooked. He had opened a can of refried beans and a can of beef broth and made two burritos. He had cooked the two tortillas on the flame on the stove. Guess he heated up the refried beans in the microwave with one of the cereal bowls. Don't know why he opened the beef broth! I checked the trash. He had taken two or three bites out of each burrito and thrown the rest away. I scolded him for cooking while I was gone. My mistake. I shouldn't have left him alone. I can't trust him. I put the rest of the refried beans in a plastic container and ran hot water in the ceramic bowl to soak since some cheese had hardened on it. Went into my office to pay bills. Ten minutes later I came back in kitchen and he was throwing the ceramic bowl away. He had broken it. Don't know how. I saw that he had fixed a bowl of cereal and eaten part of it. Probably dropped the other bowl on top of it. He always throws things in the sink. He doesn't pay attention to anything. I just can't keep up with him and never know what he is going to do next or when. I realized I needed to do something to keep him from using the stove so I will start taking the knobs off and hiding them.

~

April 4

I came into the living room and the recliner was turned over. Beecher was sitting on the floor next to it still playing his iPad. Said he wasn't hurt. It was like he didn't even know he had fallen and knocked the chair over.

April 5, Easter Sunday

Michelle fixed dinner at her house and had all the family over. Nice day with no problems with Beech.

~

April 9

Took him to the VA to get his chest x-ray. Notified the social worker. She will have the results sent over with an approval letter for the Respite Care.

April 10

Another crazy day. Beecher's not paying attention to anything I say. Keeps repeating everything. Took him to Jack in the Box for lunch. Stopped at the store to get movie for tonight. Beecher wandered off to find something. Ended up with two candy bars and some gum. Said he wanted some sweet cream for his coffee but when I went to get it, he walked away. When we got in the car, he said to take him to Vons for some sweet cream. Once we got home, he changed his shoes twice and even opened the garage door and went and sat in car. He thought we were going to Vons after I told him at least ten times we weren't. He also made an ice cream float and then changed cups. He spilled almost all of it on the counter when he poured it from one cup to another. Another mess to clean up! He's really out of it today. Frances isn't coming for a few days. She hurt her back. Boy, do I miss her! Also, this morning, I saw him heading to sit in the recliner and he almost fell forward into the chair. Of course, he had his iPad in his hands so he wasn't paying attention again. His friend Gary and his girlfriend are coming to visit tomorrow and staying the night. He is really going to be surprised at the difference in Beech.

It's now 4:00 and he's putting on his shoes again to go to Vons. He just isn't getting it. Went and sat in car again. Waited a few minutes and went out to garage and he came back in. Also noticed he had cut the top off cookie mix and spilled part of it on counter. Well, it's been five minutes and he just changed his shoes again and went out to sit in the car!

April 11

Another friend of ours, Gary and his girlfriend Maggie came to visit us from Arizona. They took us to dinner at Pin Kaow. We ate outside and it was very nice weather. Then we drove out to Lake Las Vegas. Walked around and listened to some music. At one point while they were playing "It's been a hard day's night," Beecher and I started dancing and he sang along with the song. It was a touching few moments. He was Beech again if only for a few moments. I had a nice time. Weather was still gorgeous. Went to the chocolate factory and saw Patti's friend Sue who owns the place. After we bought some chocolate, Beecher walked out and disappeared. We went looking for him. He had walked back to the car. Gary found him and we walked around for a little while longer. He kept trying to walk away again. And he wasn't heading to the bathroom for a change. All in all, we had a great time and I enjoyed meeting Maggie and spending time with Gary. I'm sure Gary was surprised at how different Beech was. He couldn't believe it had been over two years. He did say he noticed something different about him when he came to Vegas to go to the seminar that their friend Duncan was doing in Pahrump a few years ago.

April 12

Gary and Maggie left around 10 am. Gary said they would be coming back to visit soon. He gave me some money and said, "If things were reversed, I know you guys would do the same for me." He is such a nice guy. I'm so glad to have him for a true friend. He cares very much for Beecher. Well, today was eventful once again. I went to fix Beecher lunch and he grabbed a bowl out of the cupboard before I had a chance to get it. He dropped and broke it. I'm now down to five bowls out of eight. I fixed dinner while holding my breath. After eating, Beecher stood up and started to carry his plate to the kitchen and then stopped. I reached out to take the plate from him and he just let go of it. It shattered as far as the living room carpet. I'm now down to eight plates out of twelve. Need to get all plastic dishes for him! Will look into that this week for sure!

April 13

Stress free day. Beech is at Adult Day Care all day! Oh wait! I almost made it through the day. Not his fault this time. I was just heading out the door to pick Beecher up when I got a call from my friend Belinda. Her and her husband Terry were at the Village Pub to have dinner. That's where the bus drops Beech off and where I pick him up. Well, he was inside the Pub. Belinda called out to him and he kept walking. He walked out of the pub and was wandering around the parking lot. She ran out to him and brought him back inside and called me. The bus had picked him up a half hour early from the Day Care so they dropped him off at the pub a half hour early!! Thank goodness Belinda was there or I wouldn't have known and he could have wandered off and gotten hurt or lost. I was really upset. By the time I got to the pub, he was eating dinner with them! They shared their dinner with us. So not a bad day after all. I am going to give Paratransit a piece of my mind though! Most of the time it works out pretty well, although occasionally they drop him off early and other times, they were quite late, but I dealt with it. Also, he occasionally has issues on the bus, like spilling liquid from his Sippy cup (he always tried to sneak juice into the cup and I wouldn't let him taking anything but water) or getting up too soon before the driver had opened the door to let him off the bus.

April 15

Beecher had another fall today. Amy took him to the movies. As they were leaving, he stepped off the curb wrong and fell forward. Skinned his knee but he was okay. I think Amy was more upset when she called to tell me cause it at happened on her watch. It's a reminder of how we all need to focus on his safety. It's hard sometimes when we never know what he is going to do. It makes me so nervous that he's going to get hurt worse the next time.

~

April 17

Started the day off with him breaking the lamp on his side of the bed and spilling half the bottle of mouthwash on the sink and rug. He didn't bother to tell me. Just threw the rug in the wash with a couple pairs of pants.

He had another fall today at a Mexican restaurant. Getting up to go to the bathroom, he fell out of his chair and towards the next table. He went down all the way. Seemed dazed and couldn't get up. A customer and waiter helped him up. He didn't get hurt.

After dinner I made some cookies. Beecher went and got some milk and I heard him drop a glass. It didn't break but somehow, he spilled the whole glass all over the kitchen floor and inside the refrigerator. He just poured another glass and walked away like he wasn't even aware he had made a mess. I think I'm going to have to get those locks for the refrigerator. I spend more time cleaning up messes than I would if I got up every time he needed something. He fell again tonight in the closet and I noticed a big abrasion on his back. Don't know if it was from tonight or today at the restaurant or when he fell at the movies on Wednesday. Only people who have been through the same thing would understand and know that I am not making this up. You can't make these things up. These things happen every day.

~

April 18

I took Beecher to Physical therapy at the VA today. Ten minutes on the elliptical and then outside to teach him how to get in and out of the car safely. Repetition is the answer. Something we will have to work on.

Stopped at the 99cent store on way home and then to the In N Out for lunch. He went right into the bathroom when we got there. After we got our food (boy what a mess he made) he got up to fill his drink. I told him to wait until he had drunk more. He had napkins all over the place and ketchup all over his hands. After he finished eating, I told him to go wash up. A really nice young man brought me some more napkins. I thanked him. I could tell by the look in his eyes he felt compassion for me. He could see the look of frustration on my face. Beech continued to try and take my food tray and I kept telling him to wait until I was done. I finally let him take it. He almost fell when he got up. The young man looked me in the eyes again as we were leaving. I thanked him again. There are no words to describe how that young man made me feel. It was like he was feeling my pain for me. There are still some compassionate people in the world.

April 19

Every day is different. Nothing major just a lot of the same. Doesn't answer me most of the time. Very spacey all day. Played his iPad most of the day. Took the recycled can out to garage but dumped all the papers on the garage floor instead of inside the can.

April 20

Day Care today. Another day off for me! I talked to Beecher's friend, Mark Schindler today. He was in the service with Beech. Thought maybe he would have some info on any accidents that Beech might have had in the service that could have caused head trauma but he didn't know. I picked up Beech from bus stop and fed him dinner. Told him to get ready for bed and get his slippers on. He did and then ten minutes later he started getting dressed again. Asked him what day it was, and he said, "Thursday." It's Monday. Fifteen minutes later he had changed again and came into my office. I thought he wanted to show me something. I followed him out to the garage. He got in the car. I asked him where he was going. He wouldn't answer. Told him we weren't going anywhere. He seemed confused. Came back in and got undressed again. I finally got it out of him that he thought we were going to the store for ice cream. I guess in his mind we were but he never said a word to me.

April 23

San Diego here I come! Michelle and Amy are going with me. FTD education conference on Friday. Took Beech to Silver Hills nursing home to stay for five days. Minimum is five days respite. Had some issues checking him in. Didn't seem they were ready for him. More paperwork. Including inventory. No tour of the facility. Left feeling a little uneasy leaving him but I had to get on the road. Arrived in San Diego and settled in after eating at The Fish Market! Great food!

April 24

Conference started at 9:30. Learning a lot.

Right after lunch I got a call from a nurse at Silver Hills. Said Beech had wandered out of the facilities but they found him across the street! He had a roaming bracelet on but he got out the exit door which wasn't tracked to the bracelet.

They wanted to transfer him to Royal Springs (another facility that I had looked at.) They said they would call me back when they did. Got another call awhile later from the charge nurse telling me they were transferring him to a hospital and were putting him in the psych ward in lockdown.

I was shocked and upset! Just about fell apart.

April 25-28

I finally got hold of one of the nurses. He wanted me to come and pick Beecher up. I explained that I was out of town. Then he wanted my brother to pick him up as he was my contact if they could not get ahold of me. I explained that he was working and could not take care of him. He was only listed as a contact person. The nurse was very impatient with me. I was furious because this was supposed to be a locked facility. They told me he had been walking around and bumping into trays and other people. They said he was sundowning: a condition of confusion and restlessness in the evening or when then the sun is setting, which is quite common in patients with dementia. When I checked him into the facility, I explained explicitly that they needed to show him around as soon as I left, which they did not do. After numerous attempts to get hold of someone in charge; (the director), I finally found that he did not get transferred to Royal Springs because Silver Hills did not get the clinical paperwork over to them in time before the office closed. It was faxed after 5 p.m. All they had received was his physical process report. Needless to say, this ruined my time away and made me leery about placing him again in the future. I was finally told that they had transferred him to Centennial Hospital by ambulance and placed in lockdown. Even if I was to return back home early, I could not pick him up until April 28 (five days away). That was the law they said. My brother Ricky visited him several times over the next few days, taking him tacos and spending some time there with him. That seemed to calm him down. Ricky said when he visited him; all of his clothes were all over the room. He had a guard at the entrance to his room. They did let him wander around this section of the ward to let out some of his anxiety.

When I picked him up on April 28, Beecher had such a relief look on his face that he was finally getting out of there. I was astonished at the report that Silver Hills had filled out describing his behavior. "Admitting diagnosis of unspecified dementia" (not true)! They knew exactly what he had. FTD. It was on the paperwork I filled out before he was admitted. They said he would not respond when they asked him multiple questions, stares at walls, constantly pacing and walking (normal for his disease) throughout the facility, bumping into objects and other patients causing harm to others. They said he had an elopement issue.

This facility was supposed to be a secure locked facility and he had a roaming bracelet on to prevent this from happening. When I questioned them, they told me only the front door was locked but none of the exit doors were, which is how he escaped. Another issue I had was they had no authorization from the VA to transfer him to a hospital for lockdown.

Note: It took me months to get all the hospital and ambulance bills straightened out until the VA paid for all of it. What a nightmare!

All in all, since I could not do anything about the situation, my daughters and I learned a lot at the conference. The conference was broken down into Breakout Sessions. We each went to a different one so that we all could take notes and then share it with each other. This helped us all gain much more knowledge, especially for my daughters. I was amazed at their tenacity in wanting to learn all about this dreadful disease. They communicated very well with me and others and even spent some time talking with some of the patients who had FTD who attended the conference.

My daughter Michelle attended the Breakout Session on Movement Disorders, regarding PSP, CBD or FTD. Some of their studies included patients with FTD who have motor disturbances such as PSP have shortened survival rates indicated by early falls. Those with CBS have a survival rate of + or - is five to eight years. This was alarming to me as Beecher has being having many falls for a long time. Although PSP and CBD are still under-diagnosed, there are clear advances in the field. They have a better understanding of genetic and environmental factors. It was also mentioned that patients with PPA have a hard time communicating and that we need to be extra sensitive to them. Some of the suggestions and for the patient included:

- *Speak one on one, if possible. Face to face with direct eye contact is best.*
- *You don't always have to use the perfect word, alternates are ok.*

- *Use non-verbal modes of communicating, such as gestures or touch.*
- *If you feel speech is slipping away, stop speaking. Silence can be restorative.*
- *Create "awareness cards" to present to others that let them know your loved one has a language and behavior problem that may be altered due to the disease.*

Early on in Beecher's situation, he learned a little sign language in day care, mostly how to say "I Love You", and a thumbs-ups meant "yes" or "ok" and a thumbs-down meant "no."

I made "Awareness Cards" stating he had speech and behavior problems due to a degenerative brain disease. He handed them out quite often as well as I did. I even gave some to my daughters as sometimes they were alone with him, such as the movies or lunch. Be sure to include their name and caregivers phone number in case they are lost. This took off a big burden especially in public and kept the embarrassment to a limit. Although some people still refused to accept it.

Suggestions for the caregivers included strategies for modifying our own language and behaviors, such as:

- *Reducing sentence clutter: Using shorter sentences with a focus on key words, whenever possible.*
- *Reduce anxiety by allow them sufficient time and not rushing them.*
- *Yes and No questions may be easier than open ended ones.*
- *Offer choices rather that open ended questions.*
- *Supplement verbal message with gestures or movements such as "show me"*

Remember that PPA in FTD is a process. Things will change over time and what works best today will probably need revisions in the future. BE PATIENT!

Main suggestions on Living with PPA are and "What we know so far":

- *Let people know, keeping it a secret is exhausting!*
- *The process is unpredictable and frustrating.*
- *Conversations will get slower, problem solving will get harder and the memory may deteriorate. Everyone experiences these losses and grieves and that's OK.*
- *There will be a role reversal–plan for it.*
- *There will be misunderstandings and hurt feelings–that is par for the course.*
- *Pick your issues–they can't be handled all at once. If it's not important, let it slide.*
- *Keep a sense of humor. I know sometimes it's hard but remember no matter how bad a day is, look for moments of joy. They are there and celebrate them*

Amy attended the one on Behavior Changes, for people concerned with behavior changes at home, in the community and in residential care. Some highlights included:

- *Roaming is a self-soothing behavior-a symptom that cannot be changed. Get Medic Alert bracelet for them as well as yourself. The Alzheimer's Association will provide them free to the patient and a small fee for you.*
- *Punishment such as yelling or withholding something is never the answer for solving issues.*
- *People with FTD may lack the insight needed to recognize their actions as problematic, and may be unable to modify their behavior.*
- *Avoid circumstances that might trigger loss of inhibition or rude talk.*
- *Disconnect internet and supervise financial transactions if they have poor judgment of financial situations.*
- *Meet with an elder-law attorney to discuss decision-making tools to protect savings, durable power of attorney etc.*
- *Recognize that self-absorption and loss of empathy have nothing to do with you.*

- *Recognize that adolescent-like behavior that the person is "going backwards" developmentally. Modify expectations and be realistic about what they can accomplish.*
- *Confabulation – telling false stories. This is not lying, but sometimes the brain makes up when it doesn't know the answer. Don't try to correct it.*
- *Loss of sense of risk and danger or roaming in the car: Monitor driving and using power tools etc. Stop if unsafe. Have phone tracker on car or initiate driving cessation.*
- *Gorging on food: Put out food and have a safe place that is locked to hide extra food or put a lock on fridge if possible. Don't worry so much about food balance and weight gain as the person will begin to lose weight spontaneously later on.*
- *Falls – Provide assistance when patient is walking. Get help when lifting person out of bed or from a chair. Always be prepared for falls. Safety is always the biggest issue for them as well as yourself. You cannot take care of them if you are injured.*

Music is like Vitamin D and is the language of the soul. Where words fail, music speaks! It is a nutrient for the nervous system. Music is felt by the soul, not the brain. Use what they have instead of focusing about the lack of their capabilities. It can offer relaxation instead of sedation.

As I was interested in issues in advanced dementia, addressing end of life decisions and the value of Hospice, I attended the Comfort Care & End of Life Considerations which also included information on brain donation.

Some considerations included, how to:

- *Maximize the person's quality of life, keeping them safe, and methods to prevent complications and options to intervene if they occur.*
- *Modify their surroundings to enhance a sense of well-being*
- *Perform a risk/benefit analysis for all current and future treatments & medications.*

- *Talk about end-of-life considerations and choose who to include in these discussions.*
- *Make plans and develop goals for advanced care that respect the individual's wishes.*
- *Determine what services are available, including palliative and hospice care.*
- *Learn about the Hospice Eligibility criteria for Dementia. To receive Medicare Hospice the patient must be on Medicare or receiving Social Security benefits with a statement saying you choose comfort (palliative) care rather than medical care intended to cure your illness. The patient must certify with a doctor's statement that the patient has six months or less to live. They must meet all or some of the following criteria:*
- *Be unable to walk, bathe and dress independently*
- *Only able to speak a few intelligible words*
- *Be incontinent of bowel and bladder*
- *Be losing weight steadily*
- *One or more of the following has occurred in the past year:*
- *Aspiration pneumonia*
- *Kidney or urinary tract infection*
- *Recurring fever after antibiotics*
- *Pressure ulcers (bed sores)*

Persons with FTD may not appear like persons with Alzheimer's disease in their last six months of life. Memory impairment may not be as severe in some forms of FTD, which may lead clinicians to misinterpret this fact as evidence that the patient is not in an advanced stage of the disease because "they still look good." Also, the patient may still ambulate. There are barriers for people with FTD to obtain hospice services. For example, FTD may not be recognized as a terminal condition. Hospice criteria are based on the progression of the decline associated with Alzheimer's disease. It can be difficult prognosticating the last six to twelve months of life in people with most types of dementia. Signs and symptoms that may indicate the person with FTD may be in their last six to twelve months of life based on a consensus of warning sign for persons with FTD from contracted national experts in FTD include the following:

- *Stage/severity of disease*
- *difficulties of swallowing*
- *severe language impairments, immobility, incontinence and recurrent infections*
- *frequent falls*

To be prepared, learn as much as you can about the progression of FTD and complications that may arise to enhance your ability to prepare for what's ahead. Complete all legal forms early, including Advance Directives and be sure to share them with everyone involved in the care and support of the person with FTD. **Note: if your loved one is having his or her brain donated for research, be sure to inform the caregivers at the home or hospice. Provide the information on whom to call immediately after your loved passes. This is very important as the brain must be removed within 24 hours. More on that later in the book.**

On another note, find out how to get a DNR (Do Not Resuscitate) in your state. In Nevada it is an orange card that needs to be posted in the room of the patient. FYI, aspiration pneumonia is the most comfortable way to die and starvation is not an uncomfortable way to die, as the body produces endorphins.

This conference was very educational and helped all of us prepare for the coming years.

~

April 29

Frustrating day! It started with the kitchen sink being stopped up since yesterday. Frances came today. She tried to help to no avail. Her husband came after work and fixed it.

Spent over an hour trying to get Netflix working and five minutes later Beecher turned the TV off and started playing his iPad. Other things he's done today:

Gum on the rug. He pooped his pants and left them on the floor in the closet. Fell off the recliner while sitting down.

$\sim$

May 2

Amy's 38th birthday! We celebrated it at Michelle's house. More excitement today! Never a dull moment! Before we left for the party, Beecher had a root beer float and I told him no more until after Amy's party. Half-hour later as I was getting ready for Amy's birthday party, he got into the ice cream and opened another bottle of root beer (there was already one open). He spilled it all down the inside of fridge, the counter and all over the floor. Time to get locks for both fridges. Another fall from the kitchen chair. Fell against a bronze planner and bent it halfway around. Surprised he didn't get hurt. Beecher was in a good mood at the party and behaved himself. He even sang Happy Birthday to Amy all by himself! We even got it on video! It was somewhat of a whisper and he left out a few words, but he did it. Amy said it was the best birthday song ever to her. It was a fun day!

$\sim$

May 3

So much to say and so little times these days. Have to catch up on this journal soon. A lot of the same. More falls. Almost every day now. Consistently ignores my commands. Spills, spills, spills! Cleanup, cleanup, cleanup! Wonder why I'm so tired and no time to write. It's a tough job taking care of a 6'2" two-year-old. They can reach more things and they fall harder! So many bruises. Thank God no breaks. It scares me every day. At least I'm sleeping better. Worn out just picking up after him.

~

May 4

I took him to the VA for his appointment with Dr. Remson in the Rehab department to see if he found it necessary for Beecher to have a wheelchair or a walker. It was decided it might make things worse as Beecher's balance was so bad that he could actually hurt himself getting in and out of the wheelchair or fall using the walker. After we got home, I went to the VA nursing home in Boulder City. I wanted to check out the facility to see if that might be an option for Beecher. I decided against it as it was more expensive, farther away from my home and didn't seem like a good fit for Beecher.

~

May 5

Today is watercolor day. Not really in the mood but went anyway. Too much going on with Beech. He spilled chocolate syrup on rug in living room. Came home to fix him lunch and stayed home. Not taking him to watercolor anymore. It's too hard on me and stresses me out. Lots of anxiety this evening for both of us. Repeating tasks, (cleaning reading glasses, moving things around constantly, and books being picked up and down.)

~

May 6

I visited Sterling Ridge memory care home. Administrator Rachael was very nice. Thinking it might be better than the VA nursing home. They have a new wing opening up which is a locked ward. They have been renovating and should be open sometime soon. They are just waiting to get the license. Less cost than VA. They gave me a lot of info on Aid and

Attendance that I can apply for through the VA. Only problem is: I have to have Beecher admitted first before I can apply for the Pension. I was referred to Vet Angels on how to get the process started. I was fortunate to get in touch with a lady who can guide me through all the steps necessary to make it a speedy process.

~

May 8

Early morning. Up at 5:15 to get Beecher ready for Day Care. Watched him from the bed while he was taking a shower. In there about six minutes. Very slow moving and seemed dazed. Put underwear on by sink very slowly. Carried socks into closet and came back out with only one on. Went back in closet and put other one on and came back with his jeans. As he was trying to put them on and standing on one foot he fell into the shower and landed on the shower chair. He was up by the time I got to him. The shower door was partially open and he knocked it half way off the track. I've been so worried about him falling in the shower but not **into** the shower!

Next, he spilled a whole glass of white grape juice all over the kitchen floor and as I was trying to clean it up, he went and got a yogurt and managed to spill part of it on the floor. What a mess! Started cleaning the mess up and then took him to the bus for Day Care. Spent many hours on the phone regarding the hospital and ambulance bills. I made the decision to put him in the Silver Ridge Memory care center as soon as I can get Aid and Attendance from the VA and Silver Ridge is open for business. Lots to do to get him settled in. Very impressed with the home. Sent a message to Dr. Léger regarding a few issues. Told him what I was planning to do.

He said he was impressed that I still had him at home. He thanked me for taking such good care of him. I cried when I read that. Here is his response that his nurse Nancy sent to me:

Nancy,

> *Below is Dr. Léger's response.*
>
> *Seroquel: If he is really only taking 100 mg at night, then I would give him half (50 mg) for a week or two and then stop. There may be rebound agitation during the night. Have her keep in touch.*
>
> *We can certainly write a letter to support a change in the living environment. We'll wait for the decision to be made. I am very impressed that he is still at home.*
>
> *I don't think that repeating neuropsychological testing will add very much to the current management. It has been a while since a MoCA (a Cognitive Assessment Test that checks thinking abilities) was done, and we should probably attempt one when he is seen again.*
>
> *Hope this answers all the questions. Let me know if anything needs to be clarified. (end of response)*
>
> *Thanks for all you do for him.*
>
> *Hope you have a good weekend.*

So many emotions going on. Dr. Léger also said he would fill out any needed info as soon as I make the decision as to where I would place him. I feel so relieved! More calls and paperwork! On Monday, Amy, Michelle and I are going to Sterling Ridge so they can tour the home and then we are going to Lake Las Vegas for lunch. All of a sudden, I feel like I can breathe!

May 9

Another day in the life of a caregiver! What a day! PT at the VA first thing. Beecher kept running to the bathroom. Last visit finally. Home to clean up garage. Frances came today. Worked in garage for five hours sorting Beecher's tools. Got a lot done. I'm exhausted! Came in to fix dinner, stuffed bell peppers, creamed peas and potatoes. Got the peppers in the oven and went to sit down for a few minutes. Not! Beecher went out to the garage for something and then I heard him in the kitchen. Went to check on him. He had poured a bunch of white pepper into the peas. I mean a bunch! He had no answer for why he did it. Had to pour it down the sink and start over. Started the white sauce and he came into kitchen with his Sippy mug and spilled the whole glass of water on the floor! Finally got dinner done after cleaning up after his messes. Ate dinner and cleaned up the dishes. Finally got to sit down again. After five minutes, he knocked his soda off the table and then got up and spilled his water and went to pour out his ice and get some more water. Spilled the ice and water again. He's nonstop sometimes! How does anyone deal with this? It's exhausting!

May 10, Mother's Day

Beecher made me a necklace in Day Care on Friday. He was so excited when he gave it to me. He was smiling. So sweet! There is such a sweet innocence about him that it's hard to believe sometimes he can be so aggravating.

Another fall while I was in the office on the phone. Walked into living room and he was sitting on the floor in the kitchen area playing his iPad. The recliner was not tipped over so I'm assuming he missed the chair completely. The stool was moved two feet and he was resting against the wall.

He said he wasn't hurt. Thank God. Going to have to get this memory care thing done soon!

Another fall later. Just missed the chair altogether and landed on the carpet in the living room.

Amy came over and brought us Mediterranean food, some beautiful blue orchids, and a neck and shoulder massage and a hair brushing! I feel so spoiled. What a lovely evening! Tomorrow my daughters and I have a fun filled day planned at Lake Las Vegas!

May 11

Beecher is at Day Care today. My girls and I went to the Sterling Ridge memory care home so they could tour the facility. Then off to the cemetery to take roses to my mom. Then we headed to Lake Las Vegas for lunch. What a glorious day! Lunch at Luna Rosa. Chocolate martinis, great food, chocolate store for caramel apples. And then a ride in a paddle boat. We had so much fun! Great Mother's Day with my beautiful daughters. I don't know what I would do without these two girls. They are the light of my life!

On a sad note, the Day Care called and told me Beech had pooped his pants. They washed his clothes and put some other pants on him. They called it an explosion. Bet that was a mess to clean up. When I picked him up from the bus stop, he told me they had put a diaper on him. Poor guy. Can't believe it's come to this. This horrible disease has no bounds. I feel so bad for him. Wanted to cry and throw up at the same time. I hate what this disease has done to him. But he just seems to accept it. I myself have just become resilient. I don't think of myself as strong but I guess I am. The days just keep coming with new surprises every day and I just no longer fight it. It just is what it is. I have no control over it. When this journey started, I was angry, in denial and I didn't understand this disease and why it had happened to us. Not just to him, but to both of us. My life has changed in so many ways and as much as I hate it, I've learned (some) patience, compassion and to expect the unexpected. Every day is different and it can change in a heartbeat. You just keep rolling with the flow and constantly praying for a better day tomorrow. Even with all the pain and anguish there are moments of joy and I cherish each one of them as I don't know how many more I'll get.

May 12

Good day. Beech was pretty calm today. No falls or not very many messes. He ate his meals pretty good. Frances came today and played Scrabble with him.

Busy day filling out paperwork for Aid and Attendance. Got hold of the lady from vetangels.org that is helping me. She is an Angel in Disguise. Lots of pages to fill out.

She had me go to her website and print out all the pages and then asked me to call her back. She went through each page and told me exactly what I needed to do and when.

Also, paperwork for charity for hospital bill. It's been a good day. A lot accomplished! Tomorrow is Day Care so I'll have all day to finish paperwork.

∼

May 13

Day Care today. Got started early on paperwork. Got the VA Intent to file a claim filled out and sent it certified mail so I can get a claim number ASAP while I fill out the rest of the paperwork which I need to get done by June 1st or else I lose a month's pension. Also got the Charity Application for Centennial Hills Hospital finished and dropped in the mail! Yay! I am partway done!

Going to Nevada Watercolor Society meeting tonight. Taking my Symphony of Roses picture that I painted. They are giving out ribbons for the best pictures.

∼

May 14

No ribbons for me. Oh well. I should get a blue ribbon for taking care of Beech! LOL! Enjoyed seeing all the different paintings. Nothing else to say today.

~

May 15

Day Care today so I got a lot of paperwork done! Watched the movie "You're Not You" with Hilary Swank. It's about a 35 yr old married woman with ALS and the bonding between her and her caregiver. Excellent movie but cried my eyes out.

Went to pick up Beech from bus stop at Village Pub. When the bus arrived, my car wouldn't start so had to call Triple A for a jump. Still wouldn't start. Needed a new battery. While waiting we ate at Village Pub. Got towed home. What a night! Came home and watched "Still Alice"– cried my eyes out again. It was a movie with Julianne Moore who got early onset Alzheimer's at age 50. I got my sappy movies over with and a lot of tears shed–two in one day!

~

May 16

Got up early and called Triple A to come and tow my car again to Walmart. After the flatbed arrived, Beech climbed into the front seat and while looking for the seat belt he opened the console and dumped all the contents out including coins. Beech tried climbing into the back seat to help. Almost fell. Got him back into the front seat to turn him around and then helped him out. Almost fell again coming down two steps. Another reason, I need to put him in a home. He is a safety problem to me and himself. If he had fallen, he could have hurt me seriously. I made him sit on front porch until the driver was ready. Had my car towed to Walmart. I thought battery was under warranty. Not! While I was there, I got the oil changed. On the way home I stopped at Discount Tires and had the tires rotated. So, it was an accomplished morning.

Frances came and helped Beecher get his clothes ready for the Helldorado Rodeo. I'm taking him to tonight, compliments of our friend Beverly. He started getting ready at 2:00. Rodeo starts at 7:30. He made sure his General Chairman belt buckle was shined up! He could not get his cowboy boots on. Anyway, he looked so handsome and so happy. Had a good time but had to get up and down a lot plus there were stairs to deal with. But I managed with Beverly's help. Saw a few good friends: Mario, Lee Butts, Bill and Marie Seals and Skip. Had his picture taken with Miss Nevada. That made him smile! He got involved with the antics and was clapping a lot. Was good to see him so animated! Left a little early to beat the traffic. Fun night, but I know that will be his last rodeo and that makes me so sad. He was always so involved with the Elks. He was Exalted Ruler and General Chairman of Helldorado in 1995-1996.

$$\sim$$

May 17

Uneventful day. Spent four hours in the garage sorting tools. Just about finished. I will call my son-in-law Cole to come over next weekend to help me price them. Hopefully I will make enough to pay for the first month at the nursing home.

Made soup for lunch and after he finished eating. he poured the rest of it down the wrong side of the sink. Soup had crackers in it so wouldn't go down. I had a pan soaking in the garbage disposal side but instead of moving it, he just poured the soup down the other side. Stuff like this happens all the time. He just doesn't know it's wrong.

$$\sim$$

May 18

Day Care today. Got more paperwork done. Almost finished. Just need to pick up some papers from the doctors and nursing home. Hopefully be ready to mail to VA by Friday.

Sad day. My best friend Sandy texted me. Her sister Barb died last night. She was 67. Grew up with both of them since I was thirteen. She had COPD.

Not much to say about Beech today. Fed him dinner then cleaned up after him. What a mess he makes. Worse than a two-year-old! I don't know how many times I've said that but it's the truth. Left freezer door open all the way. Good thing I got up and checked. He misplaced his Walkman. Was going to listen to some music. He had it in his hand one minute and it disappeared the next. Don't know what he does with things but they disappear so fast.

~

May 19

First thing this morning after his shower, he fell in the kitchen. Saw the iPad on the floor so assuming he was playing with it when he fell. When he got up, he was very wobbly. Didn't seem to be hurt. Fifteen minutes later he was walking and playing it again and very unsteady on his feet. Later in the day, he defecated all over the toilet. He tried to clean it up, but made a worse mess. Mama Nancy to the rescue! Yuck!

~

May 20

Watched him get ready for Day Care. He started putting on his underwear before he took his shower. After he got ready, he went out to the garage and sat in car. It was only 6:10. We didn't have to leave until 6:45. When we got ready to leave, I noticed he had filled up his Sippy cup with grape juice. He can't do that anymore and doesn't seem to remember even though I've told him many times. I don't want him spilling anything in the bus.

May 21

Visit to the VA for walker training. They encouraged me not to get one for him. Said it would be more of a safety issue since he gets up and just goes. I agreed. He was very stubborn today. Kept walking off to go to bathroom and I couldn't stop him.

While we were waiting, a guy walked in and Beecher whispered " I know that guy." I asked the guy if he knew him and he walked over and said yes. Turns out he was CJ from J&J where Beecher used to work. Hadn't seen him in two years but Beecher still recognized him. Went home for lunch and made him tomato soup. He put about eight Ritz crackers in the soup. Within a minute or so, while I walked back to the kitchen to heat up my lunch, Beecher managed to get crushed crackers on the table, floor, carpet and a little in the soup. He kept trying to get more crackers. Had lots of anxiety tonight. Up and down a lot. Everything in disarray. Typically, all his toiletries are everywhere, no tops get put on anything, toothbrush is sometimes on the floor and he never bothers to pick anything up. Just leaves it and walks right by it. Clothes everywhere. Everything everywhere. Lots of trouble with remotes, both TV's and chair. Fell out of bed with his iPad while trying to get some soft music playing. He just lay on the floor and kept playing with the iPad.

～

May 22

So glad its Day care today. I need a rest after yesterday! Beecher was very obstinate this morning. I tried to get him to stop putting grape juice into his Sippy cup. Told him he couldn't take it to Day Care. I couldn't stop him. I told him to drink it before he left which he did and then, put water in the cup.

～

May 23

I made him biscuits and gravy at his request this morning. Two hours later he went to the fridge to get some yogurt. I heard him in the kitchen and when I walked out, I saw the yogurt on the table. Somehow it had shot all the way across the kitchen rug, the floor and onto the living room carpet. Don't know how it happened. Must have been when he took the lid off the yogurt. Francis came today and said he was very antsy.

~

May 24

Nothing much different today. Spent three more hours in the garage. I got all the tools in order. My son-in-law, Cole is coming over to help me price them so I can sell them.

~

May 25, Memorial Day

Cole came over and helped me price the tools. Frances came over at five so I could go to the potluck at Candee's house. Had fun and relaxed. Had some sangria and visited with good friends. I needed it. Same kind of day otherwise. Beecher fixed some popcorn, added 3/4 cube of butter. Ate about half and threw the rest away. He cannot stay on track of the TV programs. Constantly changing the channels or watches the same ones over and over and having more trouble with the remote. Drooling a lot lately. Doesn't rinse his mouth when he brushes his teeth. Fell off the bed tonight while I was gone. Frances said he lay on the bed to play his iPad. I noticed a huge bruise on the back of his leg. He wet his underwear when he went to the bathroom just before going to bed. He's been doing that a lot lately. How can one person have so many different issues?

~

May 26

Rough day! Beecher has been really antsy again. Up and down and moving things around. He turned the bed covers down around 2:00 pm. Got in bed at three just as I was leaving to go to the post office. When I got home, he was in his underwear. He had his clothes ready for Day Care for tomorrow. Also noticed the table lamp on the end table was knocked over. Don't know when that happened.

Disappointing day! Got a letter from VA saying Beecher didn't sign the pension form. But he did. I think it's because his signature has changed so much, they probably didn't realize it was his signature. Had to send a copy to them and hope they receive it by Friday in case there is a problem. It could affect the beginning date of entitlement for the pension.

If that weren't enough, I found out that Rachel from the nursing home no longer works there. She got a job at another community. Really liked her and very disappointed. Going to go look at another memory care tomorrow with Amy just to compare. It's called Sunrise in Henderson.

One of my watercolor teachers, William came over and bought some tools from me. First sale! Only $2700 more to go to pay the first month nursing home. Glad tomorrow is Day Care day!

May 27

Day Care. Got up at five and took him to the bus stop. Came home and spent three hours pricing the tools and getting the ones I'm keeping in order. Amy came over at three. We went to my friend Linda Tozzi's to look at her Casita. Then we went to the Sunrise of Henderson Memory Care to check out the facility. Very nice property but verrrrrrry expensive! Good to see a different place. Then went to Prestige memory care. Just got a brochure. No time for a tour. Tomorrow is Beecher's assessment at Sterling Ridge and a tour for him. I've decided that is the best place for the price. I'm so nervous about taking him. I hope he accepts it well. Talked to his sister Lola today. Asked her and her sisters to help out financially. She will talk to Cricket and Teresa and get back to me. So emotional! Amy and I went to pick up Beech from the bus stop. Ate dinner at the Village Pub. Fish n Chips. Yummy! Going to bed in a few minutes. Exhausted!

~

May 28

One of the saddest but most relieving days of my life. I took Beecher for his assessment at Sterling Ridge where he will be staying from now on. I explained to him that he was going to be going there instead of the other Day Care. I tried to keep it very upbeat and excited so he would be excited about it. As he was introduced to the management team, he seemed to be okay although he wet his pants when we first arrived. I told the girls that he knew how to say I love you in sign language. He gave me the sign and then to the two girls. That was a moment of joy as he smiled when he did it. We proceeded to the memory care ward where he will be living.

Everything was explained to him about the activities and dining room. Making peanut butter cookies and bread seem to spark his interest some since he loves peanut butter cookies. He kept walking away to go back to the office. Not sure what he was feeling; maybe just absorbing it all and realizing that this was his life from now on. Krista and Diana were very attentive and sweet towards him. We then proceeded down the hallway to the rooms where they were going to start filling up first. There were two corner rooms that had two windows in each of them instead of one. I noticed that the one room had a big tree outside with hummingbird feeders all over it. He chose that room. I was so excited as I thought that would be the best room for him. Krista said that would be his room and that he had first choice because he is the first one to be admitted and the first one to come in for his assessment. There is another gentleman that's going to be admitted on the same day but he hasn't had his assessment yet. They will be the only two in the beginning which will give them both a chance to get to know each other and not feel alone. Although it's a semi private room, Beecher will be the only one in his room until the facility starts filling up, which is very cool. Then they will try to match up someone that fits with his personality, maybe the guy that's moving in on the same day. I feel good about the assessment but just wondering what is going through his mind. I told him that he was very special because he had his own bachelor pad and that he would have a run of the place since he was the first resident. I told him we could hang his DABEECH license plate in the shadowbox outside his room. He liked that idea. There is a secured outside area where we can go and sit or take a little stroll. We said our goodbyes and headed home.

He wouldn't talk to me or answer any of my questions. I don't know if he was upset or just still trying to absorb what was happening. I took him to Krispy Kreme and then to Jack-in-the-Box for tacos. That's what he wanted.

While we were waiting for our food, I took his sunglasses off and grabbed his two hands across the table and asked him if he was okay. I started getting teary-eyed and I saw his eyes water as well.

I told him he was going to be okay and that we would be okay. I explained to him that this is what we needed to do for his safety as well as mine and that this was our life now. I assured him I would be there every day if I could and come and have dinner with him as well when I could. Also, that Amy and Michelle and anybody else who wanted could come and visit him.

Amy picked us up and took us to the movies to see Tomorrowland because he wanted to see it. He seemed to enjoy it as he did not get up once to go to the restroom and it was a two-hour movie. Came home and went to bed. I was emotionally drained. So glad this part is over.

With any luck the facility may open next week, Tuesday, June 2. I have to start preparing the clothes and furniture that I am moving into his room. The fee will be $2800 per month, all inclusive. Skilled nurses with a 1:6 ratio which is considered excellent.

Hope the Aid and Attendance starts the following month as I am going to need it. The Medic Alert bracelets that I ordered from Alzheimer's came in for both of us. His was free; mine was $35.

May 29

Up at five and ready to go to Day Care. As we were leaving, I noticed he had filled up his Sippy cup with grape juice. I told him he would have to drink it because he could not take grape juice on the bus. He guzzled it down and I filled it with water. As we were walking out the door with me behind him, he suddenly turned around to go back into the kitchen. I had the bottle of water in my hand to refill the cup but did not notice that he had taken the top off. Half of the water went down the front of my blouse. Just another reminder of some of the things that I won't have to deal with anymore on a daily basis.

When we got to the bus stop, I had to talk to the driver. I told Beecher to wait until I talked to him but as usual, he ignored me and got on the bus anyway. When I realized it, I stepped up into the bus to make sure he had his seatbelt on and I noticed he had about a four-inch scrape on his arm that was bleeding. Don't know what he scraped it on nor would he tell me how he did it.

I wiped the blood off and gave him a napkin to hold on it if it bled anymore. I then called the daycare when I got home and ask them to attend to it.

I know that next week is going to be the hardest week of my life. The hardest day of my life next to the day that I dropped my 16-year-old son Steve off at juvenile hall. He had been in trouble and was causing friction in our home. Tough love, it's called.

I remember the feeling of abandonment but I knew it was necessary. Beecher had abandonment issues all of his life growing up. His mother married thirteen times and he had many stepmothers and stepfathers. That's why this is so hard for me.

I hope Beech doesn't feel like I am deserting him. The last four years have been the hardest struggle of my life dealing with this terminal, devastating illness called FTD. We call it the stupid disease. The way I'm feeling right now it's -- I'm "Fucking Tired, Damnit!" FTD!

May 30

Can't believe another month has gone by. Got up early to go and help with the parking lot sale at the clubhouse. Frances came at nine to take care of Beech.

At noon, Beecher's friends from the Elks Lodge, Mario and Bobby Keck took us to lunch at Winchell's. Had a nice visit with them. Talked a little about the rodeo. Got a few smiles out of Beecher. Quiet evening except for a few spills, once with root-beer over half the floor in kitchen. Frances had just mopped the floor before she left! Never stays clean for more than half a day. Used to it now. Early to bed.

May 31

Up early. Took Beech to breakfast at Egg Works. He almost fell twice getting up out of the booth. This is the last time I will be taking him out to eat before he goes to the memory care home.

Family coming over tonight. Making pulled pork and Beecher's baked beans. He even helped me! And I made his favorite dessert; German chocolate cake. Last get together with everyone before he moves into his "bachelor pad." Amy, Michelle, Cole, Justin, Bethany, Ricky and Christine came over. Had a nice time. Beecher fell in the garage and hit his face. He was taking the recycled trash out. I just happened to follow him and found him sprawled on the floor between my car and the tables that I had set up with tools. The trash was everywhere and he was trying to pick it up. The two tables were pushed back and apart but I don't know how it happened. Justin, my grandson was just coming in the door and I yelled to him to help me. He pulled Beecher to his feet.

Beecher was up and down throughout the evening and kept changing the DVD from one movie to the next. Also, he went into my office for something and I followed him there. He almost fell into my desk where my lamp was. His balance is really getting bad. I hope I can get him in the memory care home this week before he gets hurts bad.

After dinner, he kept changing the CD in his Walkman over and over. He walked out of the bedroom into the living room in his T-shirt and underwear with his sleep mask on his forehead and his ear pads on his ears sticking on the wrong way. All the kids were still here.

We all laughed at him and he laughed too. Took pictures of him and everyone. The funniest part of the night.

Tomorrow is another Day Care.

~

June 1

As I get closer to placing him in a home, every day is a reminder of why I need to do this. This morning was another example of why. Had the alarm set to wake up at 5:15.

Beecher woke me up at 3:45. He already had his shower and was in the bathroom. Lights on with the door open. Bedroom door open. Lights on in the kitchen.

Two chairs knocked over at the kitchen table. One was resting against the sliding glass door. He had eaten his yogurt and I stepped in some of it on the kitchen floor. Light and fan was also on in the guest bath.

I tried to go back to sleep but finally gave up, plus I needed to keep an eye on him. It's now 4:30 and I don't have to leave until 6 to take him to the bus stop. He's now sitting down and playing his iPad. Guess I'll doze in the recliner for a bit. If I'm lucky.

My sister Patti came over. She bought some tools. Went to the knife store and got some knives appraised. Sold them to Robert. my nephew. Good money day!! I still have a lot more tools to sell.

Picked Beech up at the bus stop at 6:00 and came home and fixed him dinner. After dinner he kept changing the movie in the DVD player. Finally encouraged him to go to bed which he did.

Tomorrow, he has a dentist appointment at 9:30. Hope that goes well.

June 2

Dentist appointment went well. X-ray and exam. Has to go to an oral surgeon and get a tooth pulled. Will wait to have it done after he moves into the facility since he's not in any pain.

Well, the date for the move in at the nursing home has been changed to Tuesday, June 9 right after his VA appointment with his primary doctor. Very disappointed because I have been counting the days. Beecher's primary doctor is on vacation until Monday. She has to sign all the paperwork. Frances came over and brought some stew for dinner. Went to my group meeting. Good meeting tonight. I needed it!

June 3

Day Care today. Got a lot done. Shopped for new socks and underwear for Beecher. Also got a lamp for his room and finished getting the pictures ready with Plexiglas.

Picked him up at bus stop at six. Bus was an hour late. Took him to the new Blaze Pizza for dinner. Only $7! They cook in 180 seconds! Came home and watched "America's Got Talent." In bed by 9:15. I'm Exhausted!

June 4

My son Steve's birthday. He turned 51 today. Boy, do I feel old! Yes, I do have a son. He's my oldest child. He lives in Salt Lake City so I don't get to see him very often. Too far away. I certainly don't have time to go visit and I'm not much into entertaining these days if you know what I mean. Here I am still raising kids: my 60-year-old who is really like a two-year-old. I've decided I don't want to raise any more kids. The grownup ones are worse!

Took him to the VA for his blood work first thing this morning. Went well. Came home and fixed him French toast and bacon for breakfast. Seems weird that I am doing so many things for him for the last time. Last time out to breakfast and last time out for pizza Frances came at eleven. I worked out in the garage for a while.

Beecher made his daily root beer float. He always softens the ice cream in the microwave. Then puts it in a coffee mug and microwaves it again. He dropped (not put) the coffee mug in the sink. Of course, it broke. It was one of my favorite ones that said "Take me to the Beach! This is the third one he has broken the past few months that I know of. After Frances left, he started changing the DVD's like five times. He can't work the remote correctly anymore so I have to do it each time. It gets so tiring. Up and down. Then I saw him with my kitchen shears heading into the bedroom. He doesn't answer when I ask him what he's doing. I took the shears away from him and followed him to the closet. He wants to trim his rubber insoles for his shoes. I guess they are all of a sudden too big? He's only had them for about five years!! I'm glad tomorrow is day care. I need the rest!

I fixed dinner and called him to the table. He was in the bathroom getting his clothes ready for Day Care for tomorrow. He walked to the kitchen sink and spit something out of his mouth, mostly on the counter, because he never reaches the sink. Five times he tried to get up while eating to go back to his tasks. Had to tell him five times to sit down and finish eating. He finally did finish and then walked back to the bedroom with his Sippy cup. A few minutes later, he carried his Sippy cup to the bedroom again, then walked back to the living room with it. He set it on the end table by his chair and, of course, he spilled it. He had unscrewed the top and didn't screw it back on and all the water in it spilled on the carpet. Glad it was water! This happens a lot. Reminders do not work. I can tell him fifteen to twenty times a day, to screw the lid on before he carries it from room to room, or remind him to watch where he is going when he has his iPad in his hands. And the numerous times, I remind him to close the leg part of the recliner before he gets up or sits down. He never does. I can tell him 25 times a day to close the fridge or the freezer when he uses it. I can hear him from the other room as he is getting something right now, this second as I write this, and I guarantee something will be left open. The numerous times I pick up the little blue gremlin toothpicks that he drops all over the house. And the most worrisome times when I say, "Be careful, you're going to fall." And the many times, I or Frances run to try to prevent him from falling. Or how about the constant messes he makes in the kitchen, the dining room and the bathroom that create a mine field. Everything is out of place and everywhere. And the broken dishes, glasses, lamps, George Foreman Grill, etc. And the many times he has lost his wallet (which he doesn't carry anymore), the eyeglasses, the sunglasses, the remotes to the TV.

It's a guessing game every day as I spend hours sometimes trying to find a certain object, especially the remote. It's one of the only times I can get him to do something else besides making messes, and I might just get to sit down for a while and watch something all the way through. I wait for him to go to bed and I pray he doesn't wake up until it's time to go somewhere, or just hope he'll sleep in so I can enjoy a few hours of quiet time. These are just some of the things that happen during a typical day with him. He's a 6'2," two-year-old on steroids!

Another fall just a few minutes ago; this time he fell off the bed while he was playing with his iPad. He just sat there on the floor so I let him be. I just walked into the other room to see what he was up to, and he had a big abrasion all down his back. Must have done it when he fell. God help me get through these next few days until he goes to the memory care home. It's too much; I just can't take it anymore.

When I came into the living room, I noticed the TV was pushed back on one side. Don't know what happened or when.

~

June 5

Our dog Cammie would have been fourteen years old today. She was a wonderful dog and I still miss her. Beecher at Day Care today. Boy I really needed the break after yesterday. Scheduled him for Saturday and also on Monday. On Sunday Frances will be coming over. Last time for her if all goes well on Tuesday.

Got a call from Kevin at Sterling Ridge and they got their license! Yahoo! Only hold up could be if the VA does not get the paperwork to Sterling Ridge on Monday or Tuesday. Plan on taking Beecher to Sterling Ridge right after his VA appointment on Tuesday. Rented a movie at Redbox and inside was a note that said, "This movie is on me. Enjoy! God Bless." Along with two $1 bills. Nice gesture from someone I don't know. Tonight, he watched most of the movie I rented from Redbox. But then he changed his underwear while he was trying to put on another t-shirt. That was the third one since he's been home. He couldn't figure out what to do. Went to bed at ten. He was up and down five or six times, brushing his teeth twice and rinsing his mouth with mouthwash.

June 6

Day Care again today. First time he has gone on a Saturday. Went to the memory home to check it out and figure out how I'm going to arrange his clothes and things. Met with Krista and got all the paperwork signed. So that's out of the way. Picked him up and made tacos for dinner. Watched a movie and in bed by 9:30. Nothing much to report. Just normal things like spilling milk, huge mess at the table when he ate. Lots of drooling all the time. He can make a mess faster than any two-year-old. One right after another. I finally got to eat my dinner. I wonder what it's going to be like when I can eat a meal in peace, get a good night's sleep and not have to clean up after him all day long. *I think I will like it!*

June 7

I'm counting down the days. Today is Sunday. Tomorrow, he goes to his last Adult Day Care. Took him to dinner at Hot N Juicy Crawfish. Best place to take a kid because he can get as messy as he wants. Then to Nielsen's custard for some ice cream. Got home about seven. Beecher picked out the movie "Big Fish" to watch but he was up and down at least ten times. Poured out his water from his Sippy cup twice, got some chocolate milk and then put some more water back in his cup. The other times, he just kept moving things around in the kitchen and then back and forth to the bedroom and back to the kitchen. He finally went to bed at 8:15. If all goes well tomorrow, he will go to his new home at Sterling Ridge on Tuesday morning after the doctor's visit. Tomorrow night will be his last night sleeping here in our home. That saddens me. But it's for the best.

Frances came today. It's her last day with us and it was hard to say goodbye. She told him she wasn't coming to our house anymore but he didn't say anything. I left to do some shopping. I made a cookbook for her, put the picture of my butterflies on the front and his colorful bird on the back. Gave her a thank you card. He leaned over to read the card. So sad. Frances and I both cried. She was a great caregiver and I will miss her. She will visit Beech and she will remain a true friend. I'm so thankful for her!

June 8

I woke up at 3:00 and couldn't get back to sleep. Woke Beecher up at 5:30. He was ready and in the car by 6. Just as we were pulling into the Village Pub where the bus picks him up the song by Lady Antebellum named "I Need You Now" came on the radio. I've had that song on my iPhone as a ring tone from Beech for over five years. Wanted to cry. Since he no longer carries a phone, I never hear it anymore. So many changes in my (our) life these last few years. No matter what the future brings I'll always feel some sentiment when that song comes on.

While we were waiting for the bus, Beecher asked me to get his pills out. I told him he already took them. He seemed a little confused. Maybe he thought he was going to Sterling Ridge.

Today is a big day. I'll be waiting patiently all day to hear from Sterling Ridge that they received the VA papers that are required to admit Beech. In the meantime, I'll be packing his things and getting them in the car so they will be ready for tomorrow morning. Tonight, will be the last time Beecher will share our bed. I'm crying as I'm writing this. Tonight, I will tell him that he will be leaving our home for the last time. This will be the hardest thing I've ever had to do.

Picked Beecher up from the bus and took him to In N Out for dinner. When we got home, I told him he was going to his new bachelor pad tomorrow. He smiled and seemed ok. He took the trash out to the street for me. Several hours later I noticed the blue can for the recycled trash was missing. I went out to the garage and saw that he had brought the other can into the garage which was still full and left the empty blue can out by the other can. Oh well. I think things will be ok. Hope I get a good night sleep, if not, tomorrow for sure. Beecher went to bed without any problems or anxiety.

$\sim$

June 9

Woke up at 3:30 and couldn't get back to sleep. Laid in bed and prayed for Beecher and cried silently for an hour. Finally got up at 4:30. I have so many mixed feelings. Don't know if I'm feeling grief or relief. I guess it's a little bit of both. The grief part is losing Beecher. I've dealt with it for almost three years. Seeing him fade away from me and becoming someone, I no longer know. The man I've been with for 26 years is now a child who knows no wrongs. A child who stares at you and once in a while you get a glimpse of the old Beech. A child that can barely talk as his speech has pretty much left him. Communication has been a big problem. Slurred, soft spoken, missing words in a sentence or all the words run together as he tries to find the right words. And me, trying to understand him and what he wants. Like a newborn baby, he has progressed backwards instead of forwards. The blank stare in his eyes that says hello but no one's home.

And then there is the feeling of relief that this part of our journey is over. The long battle has changed its course and I am closing one chapter of my life and peeking inside my new one. Like the pages you turn when reading a book, wondering what's on the next page. The relief that I won't have to clean up after him anymore or yell at him every time he spills something or breaks my favorite dish. The relief of not having to take him in public and worry about whether he's going to bump into someone or fall. The relief that I no longer will have to follow him around the house or jump up every time I hear a noise hoping he hasn't fallen again. The relief that I will no longer have to remind him to be careful getting up from the chair or sitting in the chair. The relief that I can now watch my own TV shows uninterrupted. So many things that have changed in him will no longer be a burden to me. He will have the care he needs, and I will have some of my sanity back as I move on in a new chapter of my basically single life. I will visit him daily and enjoy only the good times with him. I will adjust to my life by taking good care of myself to stay healthy in body, mind and spirit. I'll eat the right foods, and lose some weight and get back to my dance class three times a week, start enjoying my watercolor classes once again and have time to visit my friends without worrying about leaving him alone or rushing back home so the nanny can leave. No one to take care of. No one to rush home to. So many frustrations will leave me. I will have my life back and he will be in a safe place until his time on earth is done. Amen.

And so, the journey continues in a different direction. This is called separate ways. Living together is no longer. Still married, still husband and wife but just on different paths. Took him to see his primary doctor Dr Lau, at the VA. He has lost fourteen pounds in two months. Immediately drove him to his new home–Sterling Ridge. They admitted him at 10:30 am. He seemed to handle it very well. Amy, Michelle and Tyler came to help. They hung the TV, put the quilt on the wall and hung all the pictures. Room looks nice. We sat with him while he ate lunch. Then we left and got lunch for ourselves. Then Amy and I came back. Beecher was working on a puzzle and very into it. Amy and I stayed for another hour and worked on the puzzle with him. He was fine when we left so I think he's adjusting. Long day for me since I've been up since 3:30 am. Strange feeling walking into our home knowing Beecher will never be here again. Although the silence was golden, it hurts to know what has happened to us.

~

June 10

Day 2. Went to visit him. He seems to be adjusting. He drew some pictures with markers. He did a nice one with the word love. Stayed for a bit and then left to go to the health district to get a DNR form. Came back and visited him for little while longer. He sat on the love seat with me and put his arm around me. Alexa took a picture of us. There was a mix-up of his trazodone and how many he was supposed to take. Alexa will get it straightened out tomorrow so he will sleep better. Told them to give him an allergy pill that would help him since he was only taking one trazodone instead of three.

~

June 11

Went by the Adult Day Care to thank them for the wonderful care for the last three months.

On my way to visit Beecher in his new home I stopped and got him a milkshake. When I got there, he was in the bathroom and the caregiver was cleaning him up. He had messed his pants and they had to put him in the shower to get him cleaned up. They said he had loose stools. Too much fiber. They told me he had messed in the bed the night before and smeared it on the sheets. Also, the bag of toothpicks he had in his pocket had urine in them. Because of the loose stools they didn't want him to have any milkshake. I gave him a couple of sips and that made him happy. I brought him a Zentangle coloring book and he colored two pictures while I was there. I left to go to the Brain Center to take the DNR to his doctor to sign and then came back and stayed with him for a short time. I was exhausted. Need to catch up on my sleep. Around 8:00 pm. the phone rang. It was an unknown number but when I answered it, Beecher was on the other end. Turned out it was the new med nurse at night and she said he wanted to talk to me. I couldn't understand what he was saying. But he finally did say I love you and said goodbye to me. She said he was talking about his lungs being gone? Long day again but it sure is nice to come home and not have to be cleaning up after him. Almost 9:00 so I'm going to head to bed. Going to the movies and dinner with a couple of my friends from high school tomorrow so I'll have a relaxing day.

June 12

Our good friends Curt and JoAnn have set up a Give Forward fund to raise money to help us out financially. I am so humbled by the generosity. Words cannot express how overwhelmed I feel.

I woke up this morning thinking about the comments made about Beecher on the website. How he changed so many lives during our Firewalk days. He was everyone's savior. He was always trying to help someone. He was very good at matchmaking too. Went to see him again today and he seems to be settling in quite well. He fell in his bedroom and hurt his ribs. He says he's not in pain but he had a huge bruise on his left side. He said he fell against the night stand. I took him another Zentangle coloring book and he loves it. He uses his colored pencils for it. I think I made a good decision in placing him there.

June 13

I had to go to a friend's memorial service today but I stopped by to see him on the way. Our friends Janon and Kent were there. They were one of the couples who did our Firewalk's many times. They wore their Firewalk t-shirts and Beecher seemed excited to see them. I stopped by again after the service and took him some M&Ms and some Tylenol for his side. His other friends Kim and Steve had stopped by and went to get him some M&Ms and some more coloring books and crayons. His med nurse Alexa had brought in her small iPad and was letting him use it while she supervised him. He was multi-texting as he played with the iPad and then would set it down and then start coloring a few minutes later and then start playing the iPad again. Kim texted me later and told me she was surprised at how bad his illness has become as she had not seen him in a couple years and was not aware of his condition. Dinnertime came, and I went home exhausted. Tomorrow's another day.

~

June 14

Amy and I went to my granddaughter Bekkah's baby shower in St. George. Had a great time. Got to see all three of my granddaughters! They are coming to Vegas tomorrow to see Beech.

Tomorrow is our 24th Anniversary. The Home is fixing us beef stroganoff for dinner and Michelle is making sour cream enchiladas. Michelle and Cole are coming along with Amy and my three granddaughters and we are going to have a celebration! I decided to renew our wedding vows!

Amy and I stopped to see Beech on the way home from the baby shower. I ask him if he would marry me again tomorrow and he said yes. Then he looked at Amy and said Cialis?

Beecher had once given Amy's old boyfriend some Viagra, and I guess he thought she owed him some and since it was our wedding night, (well you know). We laughed so hard and he smiled because he thought it was funny too. Amy's friend Anabelle is also a minister and so she is going to marry us. Should be an interesting evening. I'm exhausted and going home to bed.

June 15

Happy 24th Anniversary to me and Beecher! I had no idea how the vow renewal was going to work out but as the day wore on ideas kept popping into my head. I got both our wedding album and our Firewalk album out and our wedding picture. (The Firewalk album had a picture of us when we renewed our vows many years ago walking on hot coals.) Amy had brought flowers for me and the girls. At the last minute I decided to wear my wedding veil. All three of my granddaughters were there and Leah was my flower girl again and Michelle and Amy were my bridesmaids. The ceremony was beautiful. Also, Amy's friend, Anabelle did the wedding vows. Everyone was in tears. Beecher and I danced to our song and then he danced with all the girls including the staff, Alexa and Michelle and the only other resident. After the ceremony he went straight for the cake after taking off his jacket. We watched videos of our first wedding and our Firewalk wedding. Amy sang "Two Lovebirds on a Limb" by Billy Falcon accompanied on guitar by her friend Jimmy. Beecher's niece, Lisa, from Bullhead city was on her way back home from Utah so she also attended. Watching the first wedding was very tearful and sentimental as I heard his voice (his real voice) as he said the words so fluently with that deep voice and without missing a word. After that we ate the food Michelle had made and then cut the cake (actually Beecher had already gotten into that.) LOL! It was a most memorable day. I don't know if he will make another year to our 25th Anniversary, so I'll just have to relish each day and each memory I have with him.

This is a message that Cole, my son-in-law sent to me. He wasn't able to attend.

June 15, 2015

I know everyone wrote something describing your marriage. I'm calling this "unwavering life, in love." The fond memories of that first kiss. The first time taking a trembling hand and saying "it's ok, I'm here and this is really me." Although, it seems distant for a moment, you can start to feel it go from your hand to your heart. All of a sudden, worries of "the right one" becomes clear and confusing at the same time. "How can someone love me before they really know who I am?" How can I have this feeling when I don't truly know who they are?" The balance of life and love begins to take form. Once your mind and heart truly believe that the one who held your hand is true, you fall into the deepest love possible. It's the turning point of what you can deal with and what you can't, in life. Struggles dealt with passion always lose, when you have true love. Adversity has no chance, when you know the truth and the end is never the end when you believe. Love you guys SO MUCH!

Cole

~

June 16

Beecher has been in the home for a week now and seems to be adjusting okay. I finally got everything squared away in his bedroom with the TV and the pictures. Making it as cozy as I can. I took some motion detector lights to put in his room so he could see when he got up in the night to use the bathroom. Also, bought some end caps for the edges of the dresser and nightstands in his room since he still falls a lot. The lamp they had in the room was too big and it was ceramic so I bought a light weight one. I've done everything I can to make his room childproof. All the pictures on the walls have Plexiglas in them in case of breakage. Wendy and Alexa and staff (Kim and Michelle) are taking good care of him. Since he is the only man in the home and one other lady, he is getting pretty much one on one care. Went to my group meeting tonight. Always feels good to let things out.

~

June 17

Nothing special to talk about today except I picked Beecher up and we went to the dentist. Beecher had a tooth pulled and I had x-rays and also had two chips on the inside of front teeth filled. Have to go back next week for teeth cleaning.

$\sim$

June 19

My oldest granddaughter, Leah graduated from college. Attended the graduation at University of Las Vegas with the family. Came home and got ready for an upcoming craft show.

$\sim$

June 23

I picked up Beecher to take him to the VA clinic to see Dr. Turner who approves and follows up on the meds that Beecher is taking. While we were waiting for his appointment, Beecher went into the bathroom. He had been in there quite a while so I went in to check on him. He was standing in the middle of the bathroom with his pants down and poop all over his pants and shoes. I told him to stay there while I went for help. I went out to the windows where you check in and told someone I needed help immediately in the bathroom. As I turned around to head back, Beecher was coming out holding his pants in front of his crotch area. I told him to go back to the bathroom. All I could see was his cute little butt as he trotted back. Sad but funny at the same time. The embarrassment of it all! (He would have been so ashamed!) I felt so bad for him and I'm sure other patients were in awe. The staff at the VA was there immediately and they cleaned the mess up on him and the bathroom. They put a diaper on him and a hospital gown and helped me take him to the car. We never got to see the doctor but he said we could do the appointment over the phone from now on. After this day, I will always carry extra shoes, extra pants, diapers and baby wipes! The home he is staying at told me that starting next month, I could have them take him to his doctor visits on their bus with a staff member, and I could meet them there for the appointment.

❧

June 26

I went to lunch with some of my girlfriends from Las Vegas High School at Macayo's Mexican Restaurant. I still need some breaks! I visit Beech at least three times per week. He spends a lot of time coloring and playing with his iPad and his Angry Birds game. He responds to me most of the time with a whisper or gives me a sign for "I love you".

❧

June 27

Today I took him some peanut butter cookies (his favorite). He also had a haircut at the memory home. I forgot to warn the stylist that he falls a lot and he almost fell getting out of the chair. Still have to watch him every minute. Sometimes I can be sitting right next to him at a table while he is coloring or eating and he gets up so fast, he falls before I can get to him. I asked the staff if they could get him a full-size bed as the twin bed is so small for him and he doesn't seem comfortable in it. They said they would. Whenever I'm there visiting, I always check his room and most of the time all of his clothes are pulled out of the drawers and the closet. I'm sure they have a hard time keeping up with him but they do it with such grace and don't seem to mind. My girlfriend, Judy's granddaughter (29) passed away from pneumonia. Went to her funeral—so sad.

July 7

I'm getting lazy about writing in my journal. Guess I don't have as much to complain about since Beecher is no longer living at home. When he was home, I often wrote in my journal to relieve tensions I was dealing with. It gave me escape from reality, I guess. Today I had lunch with my good friend, JoAnne. Nice visit. This month has flown by so fast. I seem to have a lot more time to myself, even though I go visit Beecher a lot-- sometimes by myself and other times to meet friends that want to see him. I feel a need to prepare people before they see him for the first time since he got sick. It is quite shocking since they haven't seen him in a while. He seems to be eating well; friends bring him coloring books, crayons and M & M's. He watches some TV. I took some of our movies from home. Since they have a DVD player in the TV, I thought Beecher would be watching some of the movies, but he doesn't seem to be interested in them unless it is "The Three Stooges." He used to watch that so much, I couldn't stand it after four or five times a day. When people come to visit him, most people don't think he recognizes them. But he does; he just doesn't always acknowledge them.

Just found out that our friend Connie has a daughter who was just diagnosed with FTD. She is only 54. Connie and her husband Pat were good friends of ours when Beecher belonged to the Elks Lodge. Connie has been taking care of her daughter Michelle since Michelle's husband left her. No one knew what was wrong with her until she went to the Brain Center and got diagnosed. I told our good friend last December to take her there because her symptoms sounded like Beecher's. Michelle was diagnosed this past March. I recommended her to Sterling Ridge and she is now moving in the home here. Beecher knew her from the Elks Lodge too.

When they first saw each other, you could tell there was recognition and they stared at each other as they seemed to connect. She doesn't speak much either.

I took him for a walk outside. He seemed to like that. I do that as often as I can. It gives us some time alone and I feel he needs some sunshine. The home is starting to fill up with more residents and more caregivers. Beecher has had a few falls but nothing serious yet.

July 8

I went to the Lunch and Learn at the Brain Center. It was very informative. They talked about how music was good for patients with dementia. I took a CD player and Beecher's favorite CD's to Sterling Ridge and the home started playing his music during lunch time or quiet time in the main dining room. They got him a full-size bed. Thank goodness. I hadn't realized until now how tough that must have been for him going from a king size bed to a twin bed. He seems to be much more comfortable in the full size. Only thing is that he can get hurt on the headboard as he seems to sleep in funny positions. Sometimes when I go visit, he is taking a nap and I go into his room and watch him sleep. And sometimes I lay on the bed next to him. I can do that now that he is in a bigger bed. I talked to Amy when I got home and she is going to make a padding to go over the wooden headboard to give it some cushion.

July 10

Amy made the cushioned headboard and we got it to fit pretty good. She even set up a new stand for where his iPad plugs in. He kept knocking over the other one and we were afraid he was going to get hurt, plus his iPad didn't always get charged and then he didn't have it to play with. Amy set up the new stand and even chained it so it wouldn't fall over. She's so good at things like that.

July 14

Picked Beecher up and took him to the VA to see his neurologist at the VA Hospital (Dr. Galik). Beecher's walking is still pretty good, just have to watch him as he gets up and down as he sometimes suddenly loses his balance. After his visit with Dr. Galik, Beecher had to go to another room to get his vitals done. He fell getting up but wasn't hurt but the doctor was notified. They said he needed to have a wheelchair. They sent us to the Rehab Dept but they didn't have an appointment until 2 pm. I didn't want to drive him back to the home and then bring him back again as it was only 11 am and a long way back.

To kill some time, I decided to take him to lunch close by and drive by our old house not too far away. Took him to In N Out and then to Krispy Kreme to get him a doughnut. Drove him by our old house and since we still had time to kill, I took him to the park near our old house. This was not a good idea as it turned out to be the most horrible day of my life! Went to see the birds by the lake. All of a sudden, he had to go pee. I started directing him to the park bathroom but had to detour and go back to the car to get clean clothes, paper towels, diapers and baby wipes in case he made a mess. Thank God! He needed them. And what a mess it was! Not only was he a mess but it was 110 degrees that day and that park bathroom was so hot I thought I was going to pass out from the heat and the smell. He had poop everywhere; his pants, his shoes, all over the floor and the walls. I could hardly keep myself from falling as I tried to keep him from falling as I stripped him down to his birthday suit and tried to clean him up. There was no place to sit or anything to hold onto as I tried to clean him up.

I panicked while I waited for someone to walk in and see what was going on as I yelled at him to hold still so I could clean him up. Thank goodness I had a full roll of paper towels and baby wipes. I just wish I had gloves. The park personnel came to the door and asked if I needed anything and I just yelled that I was okay. Just cleaning up after my husband. So glad that no little boys had walked into that bathroom. I don't know how I had the strength to get him cleaned up without me or both of us falling in the bathroom.

I finally got him dressed in the clean clothes, got his shoes on (good thing they were slip on), but even that was difficult. Then I had to clean the bathroom as best as I could. It looked like there had been an explosion in there! Washed his hands and under his fingernails. (Yes, his fingernails!)

As I walked him back to the car, I had a sense of relief, accomplishment and sadness. Relief for getting the job done, accomplishment for something I never thought I could do, and a sadness that our life had come to this. As I looked into his empty eyes and held his hand—like a mother walking her child to the car, I realized he wasn't even aware of what had just happened. He is so innocent and I have to protect him every minute.

As sad as this day was, I felt proud to have gotten through this day. After this, I still had to take him back to the VA. We made it back to the VA just in time for his appointment, but after all this, they decided he wasn't ready for a wheelchair. He might fall getting in and out of it!

I just wanted to cry and believe me I did as soon as I took him back to the home and drove myself home. After loading his clothes in the washing machine, I took a shower and went to bed (after I cried and screamed that this life is not fair and what did I do to deserve this?) I had a meltdown like I had never had before!

~

August 2

Celebrated my daughter Michelle's 48th birthday at Hot N Juicy Crawfish. Everyone loved it. Always feel bad that Beecher can't go out anymore, but it's nice not to have to worry about him falling.

Starting this month, my support group meetings at the Brain Center will now be two times a month on the first and third Wednesday.

~

August 6

I'm a Great Grandma again! My granddaughter, Bekkah gave birth to Wesley! Can't wait to meet him!

~

August 8

Well, spoke too soon! Sterling Ridge called and said Beecher fell and hit his head. Has a two-inch gash on the back of his head. They rushed him to Desert Springs Hospital. Amy met me there. We were there for hours. He had so much anxiety we couldn't hold him down in bed. He kept trying to get up and go to the bathroom every few minutes. He swung the TV and almost hit Amy in the head two different times. He is so strong. After about an hour and a half, we were drained trying to hold him down while we were waiting for the doctor. We finally asked a doctor passing by to help us and he put some soft restraints on him. We were both so exhausted. They finally gave him a shot to calm him down and got some staples in his head. Amy had to leave for work. I drove Beecher back to the home which is only a few blocks away and I finally got home at midnight. What a day! Reminds me of when my son Steve was five years old, fell off the porch and busted his chin. It took me, two nurses and a doctor to hold him down while they stitched him up!

~

August 10

Went to visit Beech. Head is healing well. Brought Beech some M & M's. He split them with Michelle. They sit together at the table and sometimes paint together. When Connie comes to visit Michelle, she brings her treats and she shares them with Beecher like he does with her. So cute, like two kids sharing. I met our friends Ted and Joyce there. They were members of the Elks Lodge. They wanted to visit Beecher and had not seen him since he got sick. Beecher seemed happy to see them and he definitely knew who they were. Even got a picture of him and Ted and Beech was smiling!

Last month and this month are full of appointments for Beecher and me. Doctors, Dermatologist, Mammogram, follow up with doctor and then to the VA to see his Primary Doctor, Mental Health Provider for this Meds, VA Neurologist and the Neurologist at the Brain Center. Seems like that is all I do when I'm not visiting or stopping to get him a chocolate milkshake. At least I have some time to myself but I'm still caregiving for him, just not 24/7.

A couple of garage sales these past two months have earned me some money to help pay for all of his care while I wait for the VA to approve the Aid and Attendance Pension I applied for. Another flaw in our system is that a person has to already be admitted to a memory care home before you can apply for the Pension. The problem is I needed the money before to put him in the home. So, it's a waiting game. I also started selling everything I could that I no longer needed on eBay and Craigslist. It's amazing what I've sold. Beecher had so many tools and electronics. Thank goodness for that. It takes a lot of time to get ready to sell, but my daughter Michelle came over to my house and showed me how to go about it, especially about the postage and shipping. My house looks like a shipping and receiving department. Boxes everywhere but what else can I do. I have to pay the bills and this memory home is not cheap! Thank goodness it's a locked facility and Beecher can't escape!

$\sim$

August 11

Beecher had an appointment at the VA with Dr. Odtohan, his med doctor. Wendy from the home met me there with Beech. While we were waiting to see the doctor, a man walked by us in a chair type walker. He was very heavy set and he stopped to adjust something on the chair. As he did so, he bent down and forward enough that the crack of his butt was showing. Wendy noticed that Beecher had seen it and he started laughing so hard. I looked at Beecher and he continued to laugh so much that we started laughing at him for laughing. He got such a kick out of it! I'm glad the man never realized we were laughing at him. Whenever we repeated this incident to other people or reminded Beecher of it, he would start smiling and laughing again. (To this day, I can't forget that incident.)

When I got home, I wrote an email to one of the nearby restaurants to help raise money for FTD. TheFTD.org was promoting a fundraising event called "Food for Thought" coming up on October 8th and I had wanted to do something to help raise awareness for FTD. Their goal was to have at least one Food for Thought event in every state. I asked BJ's to be the host restaurant in Las Vegas. Since FTD is little known and poorly understood, as well as a life-altering disease for those affected as well as for their loved ones, I felt it important to get involved. There are three locations of the restaurant in the Las Vegas area. They all responded back and honored my request for the event. BJ's would donate 15% of food and soft beverage.

$\sim$

September 10

I finally received a letter from the VA saying we had been approved for Aid and Attendance. The amount we were awarded would be effective, retroactive to this past June 1st. However, the VA withheld the months of June, July & August until a fiduciary was assigned. They felt that Beecher needed assistance handling his affairs and they rated him incompetent for VA purposes! I was appalled! Like I'm not being appointed as fiduciary after being married for 24 years and I've been the spouse that has always handled finances? Really? Are you kidding me! Waiting all these months and expecting three months of payments and now they are holding three months! I couldn't stop crying and yelling. I was so upset. They did however state that I would receive our first payment on October 1st for the month of September and would continue to receive monthly payments going forward. After I talked to my VetAngels rep, she informed me to file a Statement in Support of Claim requesting that I be appointed to act as fiduciary on his behalf for VA benefits. You would think that since I am his wife that I would automatically have been his fiduciary. I have been handling his affairs for quite some time! I also listed some new unreimbursed expenses on the Medical Expense Report which would help increase the monthly Aid and Attendance amount in the coming months. I swear, nothing is very easy! Once I am appointed his fiduciary (if they decide I am capable), they will release the three months awards.

~

September 14

Picked Beecher up from home and took him to see his Neurologist, Dr. Léger, at the Brain Center. Beecher has lost 30 lbs. in the last three months. Down from 245 to 215. Dr. Léger said he is in the middle of the moderate stage in his decline due to a lot of factors. While we were waiting for his doctor to come in, I was looking a picture on the wall. It was a picture of a table with legs that looked like a cat. I asked Beecher what he thought it was and he said "a cat" too. Just before the doctor came in, Beech got up and walked back to the picture like he was intrigued by it. Then I told him it was a table with legs. When the doctor came in, I discussed this with him and he agreed that it looked like a table with legs but also like a cat. He was surprised about Beecher's speech and that he only whispers. He had him name several objects. Beecher's eyes indicated that he can no longer look sideways or down unless he moves his head to the right or left or down. The doctor recommended trying a medication that is used to treat patients with Parkinson's disease to help with agitation. It is called Sinemet (Levodopa/carbidopa). Dr. Léger stated on the office visit notes that Beecher's disease had progressed to Parkinson Plus Syndrome – a combination of PSP (Progressive Supranuclear Palsy) and CBD (Corticobasal Dementia).

~

September 15

Met with my attorney to make some changes in my will and start preparing for end-of-life decisions. Rough day thinking about that and what was to come in the near future but had to be done sooner or later.

September 20

Some of the girls and some of their husbands from our dance class came to visit Beech. He enjoyed seeing them all as he used to come to dance class with me, and they got to know him quite well. He always had lots of hugs and candy for the girls. My grandson Justin and Bethany came by also. They all had a good visit with Beecher and I think he was happy to see them. This past month, other friends came to see him. Kim, (who used to work for him and her husband Steve who also had worked with him). Mike and JoAnne, who had Certified us as Firewalk Instructors in 1994; and also, his nephew Denny from Ohio.

September 21

Several months ago, I had started selling on eBay to help pay for the nursing home. Beecher had several pairs of cowboy boots that he could no longer wear so I listed them on eBay. I got a request from an inter-ested buyer today that touched my heart.

The gentlemen's middle name was Wolf. He inquired about a pair of Aeroglide Double H Brown Western Boots that he wanted to bid on for his brother who was a trivia hound and likes to know the history of things. (For instance--this hat was worn by so and so). He asked if I would share some info about the boots and who wore them, interesting hobbies, or any stories that might go with the boots. He was especially interested in whether Beecher was a Veteran. I responded back to Wolf that indeed Beecher was a Veteran in the Seabees and that he had been very involved with the Elks Lodge for over 30 years. I explained his type of illness and the fact that Beecher could no longer speak or wear his boots as they were too hard for him to put on. I said "I'm sure Beecher would like someone to walk in his boots that cared about their significance." I also had some other western items including other boots and jackets that were listed on eBay which he was also interested in.

Wolf responded back. Both he and his brother would be honored to walk in his boots. He said they both cared deeply about our Veterans and truly appreciate the hardships and sacrifices they made for our freedom. He asked if Beecher could sign the boots or share his name with them. (He was actually looking for boots worn by a Veteran for a specific reason, there being a sentimental story behind it that he would be glad to share with me). I wrote back that his comments had brought tears to my eyes, and gave him some info about Beecher, including that his great grandmother was full blooded Blackfoot. I told him about Beecher's dedication to the Elks Lodge, that he was a brown belt in martial arts, a motivational speaker and that we had owned a Firewalk business. That he was a Seabee during the Vietnam era stationed in Greece and that his nickname was "Beecher the Preacher" because he was always trying to save someone. He had a heart of gold and he never wavered in his commitment to anybody or anything.

His response back included his sentimental story. He explained that he loved cowboy boots and wore them every day. In fact, he rarely wears anything else, even with his nursing scrubs! A few years back, he was bidding on some nice Justin boots that a mother had listed on behalf of her son who was in Iraq at the time and needed money for his family. She wrote in her listing, "Whoever wins this auction: promise me that you will walk tall and stand proud, for these boots were worn by a hero. When you put them on in the morning and take them off at night, stop and remember our troops, for freedom is NEVER free." Although Wolf did not win that auction, (he lost the bid at the last few seconds) it gave him goose bumps and he said, you better believe it, I would have walked tall and stood proud. He decided at that time to start a new hobby. He now collects military uniforms and boots (along with their histories) with a living tribute collection. Most of them are signed by the Armed Forces member or Veteran who wore them. He's always searching for cowboy boots worn by an American hero to add to his collection. He said he would be waiting to walk tall and proud in Beecher's honor. He would be humbled and honored to walk in his footsteps and to share his legacy with his family.

I responded back that his story brought a smile to my face and that it was a wonderful story. I asked him what his full name was. He said that Wolf is his legal middle name, but he goes by it in lieu of his first name. His native name is Mountain Wolf and he said that Beecher would appreciate that, given his own heritage.

He thanked me for my kindness and that the purchase was really important to him because he truly wanted to honor my wishes, that these boots be worn by someone who will appreciate their legacy. He hopes to have the winning bid. He also had bid on some other items as well, including another pair of boots and a jacket.

The great news is that he won the bids on all the items! I was so overwhelmed by Wolf's story, that when I mailed the packages to him today, I included an Elks buckle and one rodeo buckle that had belonged to Beecher that I placed in the boots.

September 26

Wolf wrote me back that he had received the items, and that he had worn the rodeo buckle every day in honor of Beecher. He put the BPOE buckle in their collection. (Neither of them felt right wearing that buckle since they were not Elks.) He said he was deeply honored to be allowed to help preserve Beecher's legacy and that it's a responsibility that him and his little brother would carry proudly.

He said, "I have to admit, I actually choked up a little the first time I put everything on."

He was overcome by a feeling of humility to wear these things that had been worn by one of his heroes. I was so touched by what he said that I sat for quite a while in silence as I treasured having met such a great human being.

September 27

The Elks Lodge put on a Potluck Benefit to raise money for us. Our friends and family came as well as people from Solera where we lived. Franny our nanny, and her husband, and the whole gang we used to hang out with and go on vacation with. Dave and Anita, Kathy and Todd, Jim and Kathy, Russ and Cindy, and Bruce. I decided at the last minute to pick Beecher up from Sterling Ridge and bring him to the event, since a lot of them had not seen him in a while. It was a nice turnout and we took lots of pictures. One of the Trustees, Beverly, and the ER (Exalted Ruler) set it up. There was a raffle and the ER won it but he gave it to us along with all donations from the raffle. There was such an overflow of love. I could not have done it without the help of Russ and Todd for helping me with Beech in the bathroom numerous times. They are true heroes! We are so blessed to have so many wonderful friends and family. So much love and support! At the end of the Benefit, I shared the story about the Boots which I had nicknamed DABOOTS and that Wolf had won the bid! I know it brought tears to almost everyone there.

~

October 2

Beecher's 61st birthday! Amy, Frances and I celebrated his birthday along with the residents and staff at the home. Amy had a cake made with the Jurassic theme and decorations to match since the new Jurassic movie had just come out.

We sang Happy Birthday and Beecher seemed happy but more interested in playing with the small Jurassic dinosaurs that were on the cake. My watercolor class and I had painted a picture of an orangutan for him for his birthday. Everyone in class took part in painting a portion of the painting and then signed it.

Since M & M's were his favorite candy, we had even included some of those on the painting.

~

October 4

Fine Arts Show today. I won best of show!

~

October 5

Another garage sale. I've been very busy! Still don't know how I have time for all of this! But you do what you have to do.

~

October 7

I was asked by Dr. Léger to do an article for the Cleveland Clinic's "New Thinking" magazine to share my story about Beecher and my experience of how Cleveland Clinic has helped me navigate the changes in his condition.

Since Beecher had become particularly artistic, they wanted to hear more about it and wanted some copies of some of his watercolors to include in the article. The article will be published in the spring issue of "New Thinking." I was honored to oblige.

Today I also attended the " Lunch and Learn" at the Brain Center. Dr. Léger was doing the presentation. He asked my permission to use a picture Beecher had painted to illustrate creativity which occasionally emerges as a behavior in FTD.

In Beecher's case it was his watercolor painting. Beecher had never painted before until he lost his job. I had started taking him to watercolor with me once a week to give him something to do.

~

October 8

AFTD Awareness lunch at BJ's. Amy and I met several friends at BJ's including Lisa Radin, my support group leader and who had written the book, "What if it's not Alzheimer's?' Several other people from watercolor as well as other friends dined at other locations to help spread the awareness and raise funds to help research.

October 12

Went to attorney's office and signed final corrections on my Will. One more thing to cross off my list of things to do.

October 19

Beecher had another fall! Got a call in the evening that he had been taken back to Desert Springs Hospital. Bruised his left side, hip and butt. Drove to the hospital to check on him. He had huge bruises but he didn't seem to be in pain. He behaved himself this time. After they made sure he hadn't broken any bones, I drove him back to Sterling Ridge and got him to bed. I laid on his bed with him for a while. I don't ever get a chance to do that because I am usually visiting during the day. Makes me so sad that I have lost that intimacy that we shared.

October 20

We got a notice from the attorney for the auto insurance company that they wanted Beecher to come into the office for a deposition on the lawsuit from the accident Beecher had July 16, 2013. They wanted to get it settled. I informed them because of his illness he was unable to do that. I had to get Dr. Léger to write a letter stating that Beecher suffers from a neurodegenerative syndrome resulting in impairment of memory, judgment and other cognitive functions. And in his case, language functions (producing and understanding speech) were severely impaired, to the extent that he could not meaningfully participate in a deposition. That took care of that!

~

October 29

One of Beecher's old friends from work (Glenn) came by to give him a massage in his room. He really enjoyed that. After I left and got home, I got a call from Lynn, the Director of the home, that I had to move him to another home. He had been having too many falls. Since they were an accredited VA home he was over the limit of number of falls. He had had 32 falls since he moved in. I'm sure some of them were not falls, but they had to count them even if they walked into his room and saw him sitting on the floor, they had to assume he had fallen and they recorded it as a fall. Since it was an accredited VA home, they were required to report all falls to the VA. I have to move him by Nov.1st. (Like three days from now!) They gave me a name of a home that could take him.

I was sick about this as I was originally told he would stay in the home until he passed. I think they just had too much staff that did not watch him properly, and he is a lot of work. In the first days of his stay there were only two residents and now they have over 30 with new staff coming in all the time who don't know his history and are not quite prepared for his disease. I went through so much to get him in this home and now to have to move him somewhere else. Just makes me want to scream! He's barely been there for five months. I've kept a log of his weight loss and at this time, he weighs 174 lbs. When he was first diagnosed in 2013, he weighed 264 lbs. He has lost 90 lbs. since. (34 lbs. in five months since he's been at Sterling Ridge).

November 1

Beecher's last night at Sterling Ridge. Amy and I bought the new movie, Jurassic World, bought him popcorn and candies and ice cream and took him to the theatre on the bottom floor to watch it. He fell asleep soon after he ate all the candy and ice cream. He didn't seem interested in the movie at all. I was so disappointed as we thought he would love it.

November 2

Met with the Director, Rowena and she agreed to let Beecher move in. I got him moved into the new home--Sachelle Residential Home. It's out by Sam's Town across town. Rent is $2800, the same as Sterling Ridge. Only one caregiver twelve hours by day and another one at night for twelve hours. Pretty much one on one I would say. Even though there was room for one more resident, Beecher was the only one right now.

November 4

Beecher's stepdaughter, Kimmie came to visit him from San Diego. She was shocked to see how he looked. She hadn't seen him in several years. It was a nice visit though and I think he was happy to see her.

November 5

My granddaughter Bekkah and her boyfriend Alex came to visit from Utah. I got to meet my new great grandson, Wesley. Amy and Leah were there too. Beecher even held the baby. It was so sweet. He held him very gently. Nice visit. We ordered pizza and Beecher really loved that.

~

November 8

I went to visit Beech. He seems so lonely. All he does all day is sit in the recliner and watch TV or mostly play with his iPad. Shortly after I got there, Beecher whispered to me that KD (the caregiver at night) had tied him up. I recorded what he said. Although Beecher whispers all the time when he does talk, he kept looking at the day time caregiver when he told me. I think he was afraid she would hear him. Whenever I went to visit him, she usually went into the other room, the laundry room, and she talked on the phone to someone, unless she was cooking his meals. I decided to take him for a stroll outside so I got him into his wheelchair and went out front and down the street. He didn't say anymore. The front porch has a gate that is supposed to be locked but I noticed that most of the time it's not. I made a point to let Rowena know as this is supposed to be a locked facility. I don't think he can climb over the gate as it is a little high and he would probably fall doing so.

Once I took him back inside, the caregiver took him to the dining room. I suggested she start feeding him at the table in his wheelchair instead of a dining room chair. The dining room table has glass over the wood table and there would be less of a chance for him to fall trying to get up. Can't believe she hadn't figured that out. I sat with him for a while and then went out on the porch trying to decide how I was going to handle this tying up business.

I called Rowena and told her. She said that it was a Velcro strap that went around Beecher and the chair so that the caregiver could use the bathroom. Since he had a lot of anxiety, he had been trying to bolt out the door every time she headed for the bathroom. The TV was directly in front of his chair but he could see the front door from where he sat and I guess it was an invitation to get up and leave even though he couldn't get far. I understood the situation that the caregiver has to use the bathroom sometime during the day, but they should have had another caregiver to watch him. I explained this to Beech as well as I could and told him he was not to go out the door. I later realized he told me that KD was the one that tied him up, not the daytime caregiver, so I was a little confused. At this point, I had no choice but to accept their answer as I had nowhere else to move him to. I felt so bad and scared for him. I cried all the way home.

November 10

Amy got us tickets to see Kenny Loggins at the Smith Center. It was an annual Nathan Adelson Hospice event and the twentieth event for Doctors in Concert, called Serenades of Life. Many of the local doctors that had musical talent, singing, playing piano performed. Kenny Loggins was the guest performer! Amy's friend Stephanie also went. Kenny came out to the audience and Stephanie sang with Kenny. It was so much fun and a great evening. I wish Beecher had been able to go. He always loved Kenny Loggins.

November 12

Amy and I went by to visit Beecher for a bit. He seemed happy to see us. Took him a chocolate milkshake and made him some peanut butter cookies. He always loves that. It's harder to get over to visit him as this home is much farther across town that the other home. Some days I just can't get up and make the trip. It's getting harder and harder to watch him disappear from my life. He's really become an invalid and it's so hard to see it happen to him.

November 15

Michelle and her best friend Andrea and her mom Ruth came to visit Beecher. It was a nice visit and he seemed to enjoy the company as it's so lonely at the new home since he is the only resident there. I don't much care for the caregiver. She doesn't seem to be very verbal about anything. She doesn't do any activities with him. I try to entertain him as much as I can, playing some of his favorite music and helping him paint again. He's painting a picture of a reindeer for our Christmas card this year. It's coming out good, but he paints very slowly these days. At least he's still interested in it.

~

November 16

My attorney invited me and all of his clients to a celebration of opening his new office. One of the singers from the Jersey Boys, Travis Cloer, who plays Frankie Valli entertained us. Dinner, music, wine and a great event!

~

November 19

Dr. Léger has suggested starting Beecher on the new medication called Nuedexta. He would have to have two EKG's done (once before starting the medication and then about two weeks after starting the drug) to make sure there has not been slowing of the heart since he is already on multiple medications. The medication is expected to help with agitation and has been shown to reduce behaviors such as the constant "getting up and wandering" and being "up and down" all the time. It is usually very well tolerated. I had to set up the appointments with Transportation scheduling to take him to the Michael O'Callahan Medical Center where it has to be done. More appointments! Oh well, at least it should help!

~

November 23

Not a good day! I was eating a caramel and my bridge broke. I can't get a new one because it broke off from the tooth. Like I needed this!

~

November 24

Had several more craft shows. Glad to have the extra money. Wish it was extra. Just helps pay the bills. Beecher's NA Sponsor, Raz, came by to visit him. He also had not seen Beecher for quite some time. He was shocked to see the decline. He and some other recovered addicts auctioned off a NA gold pendant that Beecher bought many years ago and he gave me the money from that. Boy did that help. Every bit helps. Beecher recognized him immediately as he does everybody. He doesn't always acknowledge them but I could tell Beech was happy to see him. I sometimes wonder what is going through his mind, whether he's embarrassed at his situation or just accepts it. It's so hard to tell. I just feel so much sorrow at how this disease has affected him, his personality and his speech. It's devastating, to say the least.

~

November 26

Michelle decided to have Thanksgiving dinner at her house. I picked Beecher up from the home and took him with me. It's getting harder to get him in and out of the car. Once I got to Michelle's, Cole came out and helped me. Beech is so unsteady on his feet. Cole was so sweet by helping out when Beecher needed to use the restroom. In all the sadness, I am so happy and lucky to have such an amazing family. Had a great time and I think Beecher enjoyed getting out and seeing everyone, including their dog Frisco who sat on his lap most of the time. I think Frisco licked up every spill. LOL! And there was a lot! On the way home, Beecher kept looking at the street signs like he thought maybe I was going to take him back home with me. That was tough. Wish I could have. I have a feeling this will be his last Thanksgiving with us.

~

November 30

Went to the dentist. They said I would need a partial to keep my teeth from moving. Just sick about this.

~

December 5

The Fine Arts Club had a Christmas party at the Village Pub. It was nice getting out to socialize.

~

December 12

Annual Christmas party at the Solera Club House. Fun but not the same without Beecher there. We always went together.

~

December 13

Amy and I picked up Beecher and took him to the Christmas laser light show at Sam's Town. They have it every year and we had been to it many years ago. By this time, Beecher had a wheelchair so it was easy to push him around. He was fascinated by the lights. We ate at Willy and

Jose's Mexican Restaurant. Beecher sure gorged down the food, chips and dip, beans, burritos, and ice cream. Amy's long-time friend Stephanie Calvert, female singer from the rock band "Mickey Thomas Starship" came down and joined us. We had a lot of good laughs and it was so good seeing Beecher have so much fun with the food. Beecher had taken me to Willy and Jose's 26 years ago and then afterward walked over to Roxy's Lounge where he proposed to me. We had pictures taken of him and Santa. It was one of the best times I'll always remember with him.

December 18

I sent a note to Dr. Léger through My Chart (a way of communicating with the doctors for non-emergencies instead of waiting for a phone call back). I addressed two issues with Beecher. #1–weight loss and #2–bed sores. Dr. Léger responded back. He stated the weight loss was due to it taking Beecher longer to eat, so he is unable to consume as much as he used to and the fact that he has less access to sweets. As to the bed sores, the doctor advised me to continue the assessments of the sores through the VA pressure sore specialist. He indicated gel pads where he sits; sofa, arm, chair and table would be helpful. He thanked me for the Christmas card I sent him and said that Beecher's art remains astonishing.

December 19

My brother Ricky's annual Higgins Holiday Happening party. Nice time. Stayed the night so I wouldn't have to drive home which would not have been good after the few drinks I had to unwind from the last few weeks.

December 25

Christmas dinner at Michelle and Cole's. Picked Beecher up again and took him with me. Beecher did very well again. Amy gave him an Angry Bird hat and he wore it most of the time. I also took our old Christmas hats we used to wear and he liked that too. He got lots of presents and enjoyed opening them. It was so fun watching him open them and creating some more memories. He's so docile now and doesn't let much bother him. He is like a sweet little boy.

When I took him back to the home, the Director's husband gave me a note saying I had to find a new home for him. He said they didn't have any caregivers and that the one that was there was moving back to the Philippines. I had until January 16th to find a new home again. Can't believe it! What a thing to do to someone on Christmas Eve! I didn't like them anyway and I don't think Beecher did either. What a sad way to end the year and possibly my last Christmas with him. Wish I could just take him away somewhere on a deserted island and let him just roam wherever he wants to and live out our life there with no worries.

December 27

My sister-in-law, Christine came to visit Beecher. She had not seen him since a few days before he went to the first memory care home. She stayed for a while and we got a chance to talk for a bit. She knew Beecher before I met him. Beecher had actually introduced her to my brother Ricky. They got married the same year we did in 1991!

December 30

My grandson, Zech came down from Utah and to visit his Grandpa Beech. He had not seen him in a couple of years. He was so shocked and upset to see him like that. He told me he felt guilty that he had not visited and he wished he had known how bad he was. He cried out on the porch and apologized for not visiting sooner. I felt so bad for him but he still had a nice visit with him. Afterwards, he took me and Amy out to dinner at Hot N Juicy Crawfish. It was really nice seeing him as I don't get to see him enough.

The life of a caregiver is really not an easy one. Every day is a challenge. As this year ends, I recall several incidents that I didn't record in my journal.

One day after taking Beecher to the doctor, we stopped to get him a haircut. As I started to pay at the front desk, the front door opened. Beecher walked out. I yelled at him to stop and wait for me, but he continued on his way, ignoring my command. Fear set in and my thoughts were to stop paying and walk out after him, (leaving the clerk to think I might not come back and pay), or do I go after him so I don't risk the chance of him wandering off somewhere or getting hit by a car in the parking lot." Of course, my first instinct is his safety. So, I go with that, and walk out and bring him back in and tell him to sit until I'm finished paying. Am I embarrassed? No, not for me, but for him. His brain no longer filters ordinary situations. He no longer knows right from wrong. Is anyone aware of this? Do people feel sorry for me or for him or both of us? The constant blank stare or the mask as they call it is predominant most of the time. The look of innocence in his eyes, which says "hello" but nobody's home. The man that I married almost 25 years ago is now replaced with someone I no longer recognize. What I'm left with are the memories of days gone by.

When did I start feeling so heartless? Is it appearing hopeless to others? Well, they have not walked in my shoes. I'm not making excuses: this is the reality of this disease. The many times I walked out of my house, away from him, as he spilled soda all over the kitchen floor, the cabinets and into the silverware drawer for the third time that day, or the day he broke my favorite dish. I wanted to escape and never come back. I feel like such a bitch sometimes. The reality is it is maddening, and the days are endless in the life of a caregiver. The decisions that a caregiver has to make are continuous. Things that seem so simple are no longer simple any more.

Many months ago, when Beecher had to give up driving, I had to stop him from pumping gas in my car for me. He enjoyed doing that for me, but he kept breaking the cap off inside and I was afraid I would end up losing the cap. I had to take that pleasure away from him. When did decisions become so hard?

The many daily frustrations do not compare to the selfless actions I sometimes have to make to survive my day without giving up, throwing in the towel, or running down the track near my home and never coming back.

There is no one to tell me how to do this. There is no one to take care of the caregiver. 2015 was the toughest year in my life as I struggled with Beecher's FTD disease. Not knowing when this nightmare disease would get the best of him, I cherished each day, as tough as it was sometimes. I watched my beloved husband change into a person I no longer knew but got an occasional glimpse of him through his smiles and sometimes a gleam in his eyes. He always seemed to be aware of what was going on around him and he always recognized me, family and friends even though he didn't always acknowledge us. Sometimes he even tried to wink at me. His eyes lit up when I brought him his favorite chocolate milkshake or peanut butter cookies. I often think of that day at the VA when he laughed so hard at the man's butt crack and whenever I repeated this incident to other people or reminded Beecher of it, he would start smiling and laughing again. (To this day, I can't forget that incident.) Thank goodness for humor!

As 2016 rolls around, I am thankful for the times I was blessed to still have him in my life, and I will always cherish the memories he blessed us with.

CHAPTER 6

2016—THE YEAR OF THE MONKEY

NEW HOME & END OF LIFE

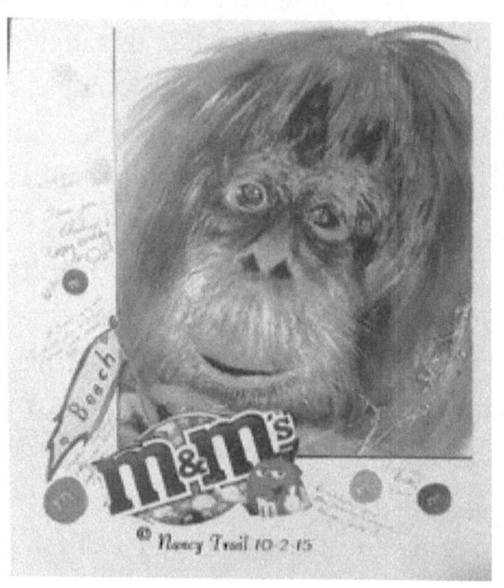

"Year of the Monkey"
By various watercolor artists in our art class.
"Monkeys are often perceived as small and powerful
but they show that a person has many friends. Sometimes I feel like I just
want this monkey off of my back!"

January 2, 2016

Found a new home for Beecher! TLC–True Loving Care. Moved Beecher to the new group home today. The director there, Francesca is so sweet. I think he will be happy there. I really like the Director and they seem to have really nice caregivers. The home is very nice and spacious and very homey and it is only 15 minutes from my house. I think this one is a keeper. I can't stand the thought of having to move him again. Keeping my fingers crossed big time! The home is $2600 which is lower than the last two homes but the VA will lower the Aid and Attendance and will end up costing me the same. Oh, well.

January 9

Francesca called and told me Beecher had an incident the night before. Went to bed for a while and caregivers heard a crash. Beech had locked himself in his room and broken a picture and was throwing a heart paperweight that one of the caregivers at the first home had given him at the dresser. When they finally got the door open, he was sitting on the floor and had stepped on some glass and had a small cut on his foot. He also hit his eyebrow on the front of his bed. Francesca said we needed to get him some meds to calm him down. I told her I would get ahold of the doctors and see what they would do. Three moves in a year and a half. Guess it's too much for him as well. Poor guy.

January 10

Because of Beecher's incident yesterday, Francesca had to make an incident report and see if his doctors would change his meds to help with anxiety. Francesca said Beecher is very restless and becoming incontinent. He's eloping, twice in the early evening. He likes to layer his clothing and sometimes he gets naked, in minutes while sitting with everyone in the living room. He gets assisted to go to the bathroom every two hours. Sometimes he stands up and starts peeing while walking. He needs to be on diaper pull ups for safety because he walks on a wet floor and falls. Sometimes he's not steady walking. Sometimes he's found sitting on the floor in his room with all his shirts, socks, and other clothing on the floor and he's playing with them or urinates or defecates on them. He needs to have a breakthrough med to control his agitation, anxiety, and restlessness.

∼

January 11

A Moment in Time! What a wonderful day visiting Beecher. My friend Belinda and I went to visit him after dance class. He recognized her and even put his arm out to her. She gave him a bag of chocolate covered pretzels and he ate half the bag. After he ate lunch, I asked him if he wanted to take a walk outside in the back yard. He got up right away. We walked him out to the patio and once we got in the sun, he turned his head up to the sky and closed his eyes as if he was taking in the sun rays and truly enjoying it. When he opened his eyes, I asked him if he was doing okay. He looked at me and put his arms around me and gave me the biggest hug I've had from him in years. He did this, five more times, and I just reveled in the warmth and sincerity of his hugs. It was like he was telling me everything was okay and I think he enjoyed the hugs as much as I did. I asked him if Belinda could have a hug and then he hugged her.

We walked him around a little more and then took him back inside as he was starting to shiver because it was a little chilly outside. Belinda went and got his red blanket and put it around his shoulders. She had some crazy jelly beans with a lot of different flavors, or should I say "odd flavors," like dirty socks, grass, baby wipes, barf, dog food etc. She gave him one, and he closed his eyes like he was trying to figure out if he had a good or bad one. We never did find out because he didn't spit it out. Then he whispered to me that he wanted a chocolate milkshake and I told him I would bring him one next time I came. He seemed very relaxed and then he put the recliner back and just started staring and smiling at me. I was so surprised at how much he was smiling that I commented to him that he sure was smiling a lot today and that I loved it when he smiled. I then asked him to give me the I love you sign. He even smiled bigger. Then I asked him to give Belinda the sign and he did as he looked at her. Then he looked back at me and continued staring at me in a way that was like his old self. He just seemed caught up in the moments and he was his old self again, except for speaking. He started to give me the love sign again, but it ended up being the middle finger! We started laughing so hard and he smiled bigger. Then I reminded him of the man at the VA when we saw his butt crack, and he smiled even bigger, almost a laugh. I haven't seen him like this in so long. It was as if he truly enjoyed the conversation and loved every minute of it, as I know I did. It was absolutely remarkable. It was one of the best days I've had with him in a long time. I felt his love and I know he felt mine. We were one for a while and I will always treasure this day. I think he truly is happy at this new home. Maybe his anxiety is starting to settle down.

January 12

Went to a high tea at a friend's house, Judy from my dance class. Nice to get out and mingle with my dear friends. Red hats and potluck. Had a great time!

January 14

Dr. Léger responded to my request for additional meds for Beech by increasing his 100 mg Trazodone to two tablets in the morning. Beecher was just taking one. He will continue to take a 300 mg Trazodone at night to help him sleep.

~

January 17

On my visit to see Beecher today, I noticed his feet and ankles were swollen. The director at the home said it was edema. It is common with all the weight loss and his blood pressure has been lower. He also sits most of the day. She will monitor him for the next few days and let me know the results. Left a message for his doctor.

~

January 18

Dr. Léger's office responded back to me in regards to the swelling. They said, in his case, prolonged sitting is most likely the cause. The doctor recommended putting a pillow under Beecher's legs when resting to keep the feet in a higher position that the rest of the body. They also suggested elastic stockings; the pressure they exert on tissues can help prevent the accumulation of fluid in the legs. Also, exercise can help. This should help until he sees his primary doctor in March.

~

January 19

Great day! Got a letter saying our lawsuit from Beecher's accident in July 2013 has been dissolved with prejudice which means she can't ever come after us with a claim. Shut case! So glad to have that off my mind!

Took a free drawing class at Michael's tonight. It was fun and I learned a lot. Great instructor!

～

January 20

Another great day! Went to my oncologist. She said I only need to see her once a year now and I can go off the Tamoxifen! Went to visit Beech. Michelle, my grandson Tyler, and Frisco, Michelle's dog came too. Had another nice visit. Got hugs from Beecher and lots of smiles. It's amazing how he knows everything that's going on and understands so much.

～

January 21

Amy took me to see the show "Shen Yun 2016" at the Smith Center. Awesome and wonderful. A great evening!

～

January 31

My old boss Grant and his wife came to live with me for a few months. They needed a place to stay and I thought I could use the company and the extra money for rent as well.

～

February 1

VA appointment today. We were at the VA for three hours seeing Beecher's mental health provider. Change of medicines. No accidents until I got him back to the home and he fell getting out of the car. Down to the ground in one second.

He got out of the car so fast, I didn't have time to get around to the other side of the car. He never listens when I tell him to wait. Not hurt, thank God.

I had to run into the home to get one of the caregivers to help me get him up. I waited until Beech ate lunch before I went home. He got something stuck in his tooth. I noticed he was pretending he had a piece of floss in his hands and pretended to floss so I got out a piece of floss and flossed for him. That was weird.

~

February 3

Grant and Alex went with me to visit Beech. He fell again and has a big cut over his right eye. He ate all the yellow curry I took him. Amazes me how engaged he is lately. Said the word yes and another time nodded no. He asked for water today. Whispered it.

~

February 5

It was an interesting visit with Beecher today. I got so many smiles and responses from him shaking his head no, saying the word yes and asking for a shower. I also asked him if he was mad at me because I'm home and he asked me to take him home. I said no I couldn't.

That about broke my heart. I've had more contact with him lately than I've had in several years. His eyes followed me when I walked into the kitchen to get some Kleenex at the island. He was also blinking his eyes as if to wink at me.

He also asked me if he could make sex.

What a memorable day! He was definitely in a good mood. What a change in him. Would like to hope its permanent, (wishful thinking), but you never know from day to day what he will be like.

~

February 10

Frances came with me to visit Beech. Grant and Alex met us there. We took him out to the back yard and Grant and Frances helped trim his mustache. She's always good with Beecher and he really likes her. It was a nice day out so we spent some time outside. Michelle and Tyler came by also. I got some great hugs from Beecher again. While he was standing up, I asked him if I could have a hug. When he did, I told him I really loved it when he hugged me, and he looked into my eyes and he hugged me five more times! I really treasured them. He also hugged Michelle and Tyler. So glad we took pictures!

February 14, Valentine's Day

Amy and I went to visit Beecher. We brought him some Valentine cards and a teddy bear and some other little goodies for him to play with. Amy also got him a tie-dyed teddy bear. Michelle, Cole and Frisco came by too. Beech was in a real good mood. Boy, I love seeing him like this!

February 19

Went to visit Beech by myself. He was in a quiet mood today. Smiled when I said "snot funny" when he blew his nose. He always said that to little kids when they had snot on their noses. I told him a friend was coming to visit him from Arizona soon. I asked if he knew who that was and he whispered Gary Hynes, his best friend from high school. Beecher finished painting his picture of the rabbit today that he's been working on for quite some time. I have a feeling this will be his last painting as he has a hard time holding the brush. It was a good visit.

February 22

Beecher's niece, Lauran, wanted to see him, so my daughters and I made plans to take Beecher out for part of the day to meet up with her. We went to a Pizza place. Beecher was really happy as he doesn't get to eat pizza at the home. Lauran had a hard time dealing with it because she had not seen him in a long time and it was a shock to her seeing him that way. But she handled it and we all had a great time.

February 23

Visit to Dr. Léger. Beecher's weight is now 184 lbs. He has lost 73 lbs. in the last year. Took him off the newest med. Noted that Beech had made several attempts to leave the home but caregivers got to him and brought him back in. At this time, Beecher walks with assistance and sometimes two caregivers. Also incontinent for quite some time. He is still feeding himself but has increasing difficulties with utensils, particularly in loading. Some choking episodes, generally from putting too much food in his mouth. Exam showed him alert but no speech output today. He can express emotions facially and with a thumbs-up. He understands and obeys simple commands. Finger movements were slowed and foot tapping slowed. His strength was grossly intact. Doctor can't believe how strong he still is. Tendon reflexes are reduced.

He is fully dependent on all his ADL's. I talked to the doctor about donating Beecher's brain. He is an organ donor. He would not very likely be able to donate his other organs since he will probably die in the True Loving Care home and not a hospital. The doctor will get me in touch with someone to start the proceedings for the brain donation. Also talked about the use of a walker. Set Beecher up for Physical Therapy appointment for March 25 at the Brain Center.

February 27

My best friend Sandy and I went to visit Beech. She hadn't seen him in a while. He seemed happy to see her. We sat and talked with him for a while and then we left to go celebrate our belated birthday lunch from last October. We both have birthdays in October and always get together.

February 28

My sister-in-law Christine and I went to see the play "To Kill a Mockingbird" at the Judy Bayley Theatre at UNLV and also had dinner at a Mediterranean restaurant nearby. Christine had never read the book. It was a great play with great actors. Nice spending time with her as well.

February 29

Visited Beecher for a short time today. He was quite animated today. He often follows me with his eyes wherever I walk. The dining room/living room is quite open and most of the residents stay in the living room area. Today Beech was making some funny faces and sticking his fingers in his ears, so I did the same back to him and he almost laughed, but it was mostly a smile. He copied whatever I was doing. So fun to see him like that.

March 1

Grant and Alex are staying with me for another month. They help a lot around the house and Grant often accompanies me on Beecher's visit to the VA. He helps getting him in and out of the car. I go to visit Beecher about every other day now. I always take him a chocolate milkshake and make him peanut butter cookies. He always shares them with the other residents and the caregivers. I'm seeing more and more of a decline as his hands are starting to become more rigid and he is having a harder time playing with his iPad. His right leg turns in and he has a harder time standing up and usually needs two or more people to help him. Getting him dressed is also a chore. I generally trim his toenails and fingernails every few weeks. They grow so fast! He seems to like the attention, especially when I rub lotion on them and massage them.

~

March 13

Beecher's best friend Gary and his other friend Jim came to visit him Beech from Arizona. Gary's wife, Sherry had made some tacos for Beecher since she knew how much Beecher loved her tacos. She packed them in a cooler so they would keep until they arrived since it's a five-hour drive. We decided to take Beecher to the park close by so they could have some private time and the weather was very nice. Amy went with us. Beecher recognized Gary right away and from the look on Gary's face I could tell it was going to be an emotional day. As we were walking out, I asked Beecher if he wanted to give Gary a hug and he stopped, turned to him, and gave him a big hug. I know Gary was surprised but happy that he did. I realized he might never get another one. We loaded up the wheelchair and off to the park we went.

Once we got to the park, they helped me get Beecher into the wheel-chair. We found a nice picnic table and ate our tacos. Beecher was in heaven. At one point, I asked Beecher to give Gary the "I love you" sign but he couldn't quite get his fingers to work right. I told him to give Gary the middle finger and he automatically stuck up his middle finger. Gary responded with "He does remember me!" We all laughed so hard, including Beecher! Gary broke into a gut laugh like I've never heard before! The look of surprise and the smile on Beecher's face was price-less and I thought Beecher was going to laugh out loud! I took a picture of that face so I could remember that look. I'm sure it is one I'll always remember. The grin on Beecher's face was priceless and the laughter he brought us of that day will be etched in my memory forever and I'm sure in Gary's as well. What a wonderful day for all of us. It was hard for Gary to say goodbye because he knew he would never see Beecher again. I know he felt bad that he hadn't been able to visit him before he got so sick, but I told him I will always treasure that day and I know Beecher enjoyed the time and the laughs and to remember the memories because that is all we have once they are gone. Whenever I feel really sad, I look at the picture that I put on my refrigerator of Beecher laughing to remind me of that day.

March 25

Francesca drove Beecher to the Brain Center for his Physical Therapy and I met them there. Not much to report. Feeling that it's too much just to get him there and back and I don't think he can do most of what they want him to do.

March 27, Easter Sunday

I haven't made as many entries this month, just too tired when I get home.

Picked Beecher up and took him to Easter dinner at Michelle's house. Amy got him some bunny ears and put them on him. Got a lot of laughs and we all had a good time. He especially loved the chocolate bunny I gave him. He even read (silently) the card I gave him. Still visiting him as much as I can and attending my group meetings at the Brain Center. It's so important to keep my sanity. I'm feeling that time is running short for him.

~

March 28

My friend, Belinda went with me again to visit Beech. He was in a good mood. He didn't eat much. He has a hard time with the utensils. The caregivers feed him most of the time and when I'm there I feed him myself. Afterwards, Belinda and I went to lunch.

~

April 2

Another night out with Amy! This time she got tickets to see The Righteous Brothers at Harrah's! We even got backstage passes!

Bucky Heard is the new singer that replaced Bobby Hatfield who died in 2003. Bucky has a style of his own and a great singer. Bill Medley sang "Unchained Melody" to honor Bobby. It was a night to remember and we even got pictures taken backstage.

Bill Medley is such a nice guy and so personal. I'm so blessed to have so many musical memories in my life, especially now with so much sad going on. Grant and Alex moved out the last day of March. Nice to have my space back.

~

April 5

VA visit to see if Beecher could get a walker. They gave him one but I don't think he will be using it. When we got back to the home, I tried to get him to use it, but he just tossed it aside as he was walking. I'm afraid it will be more of a hazard.

~

April 13

The article in the New Thinking magazine came out. It was a real nice article. It was titled "Art Expands as the Mind Degenerates." Dr. Léger included information about FTD and PPA (Primary Progressive Aphasia) which Beecher was diagnosed with early on. He explained that FTD is the most common form of dementia in people under the age of 60 and it affects the frontal and temporal lobes of the brain, which are areas associated with organizational ability, self-control, emotional responsiveness, judgment and language. People generally develop major changes in behavior and personality which Beecher exhibited in the early stages of his disease.

The article also explained how Beecher became passionate about watercolor and painted several pictures in just one class each week. He said that art is a therapeutic way for him to channel his obsessiveness and because of brain changes, some patients developed new artistic abilities, just like Beecher did. The article also included several pictures of Beecher's watercolors.

I stated that the Brain Center and Dr. Léger helped me understand what was happening to Beecher so I didn't feel alone with a disease I had never heard of. With their support, I learned how to manage his condition.

∾

April 17

Beecher's friend and NA sponsor, Raz, came by to visit Beecher. I met him there and they had a nice visit. I think Beecher was glad to see him. Amy also met us there and at one point, Beecher had tears in his eyes. Not sure what brought that on, maybe just seeing Raz. There is a part of him in there that still has emotions.

∾

April 20, Red Nose Day

My friend Belinda and I went to visit Beecher. It was Red Nose Day. Belinda brought some red noses and we all put them on. Beecher was so funny and we got a lot of laughs!

April 21

Singer Prince died today. So sad; the world is mourning.

April 27

Beecher's appointment with Dr. Odtohan, his mental health doctor at the VA. Francesca drove him there and I met them there. Beecher was very distant and non-communicative most of the time. Wouldn't respond to anything we asked him. Played with his iPad some but not as much as usual. Seemed a little sleepy or out of it today.

I usually visit Beecher at least three times during the week and most Sundays. Sometimes I stay and eat with him since its family day. I love the caregivers and the patients there. They are all so friendly and I always stop and talk to all of them. The caregivers often make special Filipino food and feed me when I'm there. They know how much I love their food. Of course, I take food to them as well. It's one big happy family there and it feels so homey. I'm so glad to have Beecher there where I feel he is truly loved. One of the caregivers, Diane, takes extra special care with him. I often find her sitting next to him when I arrive. She is hard to understand sometimes, but I feel a great love between the two of them as she is the only one that can really manage him well and he trusts her.

May 2

My daughter Amy's 39th birthday. Michelle threw a party for her at her house, Hawaiian Style. Lots of picture taking. Afterwards, Amy and I went by to visit Beecher. He was in a good mood and he even spanked Amy. You could tell he thought that was funny.

May 8, Mother's Day

Michelle's husband Cole made lobster and artichokes for dinner for everyone including Amy, my grandson Justin and his wife Bethany. Afterwards, we all went bowling! What fun! Haven't done that in years!

May 14

Visit to Beecher today. One of the residents of the home, Dan, told me he walked over to Beecher and shook hands with him and introduced himself. After he shook hands, he saluted him and Beecher saluted back. Dan knew that Beecher had been in the service and Dan also had been in the Marine Corps. Great connection and response from Beecher.

May 15

Bekkah, my granddaughter, and my great grandson, Wesley, came to visit Beecher. We all had a nice visit with them. Beecher loves little babies and especially his grandkids.

May 16

Took a day off and went to lunch with my girlfriends from high school at The Yard House at Town Square. So nice to chill and relax and talk about old times!

~

May 21-22

Took a drive out to Pahrump which is about 45 minutes away. My good friend Connie invited me to stay the night and go to dinner. Her daughter has FTD also and once stayed at the same home as Beech at Sterling Ridge. It's weird that I never heard of this disease before and to find out my friend's daughter had the same disease. Hard to comprehend to say the least for such a rare disease.

~

May 27

Got a call from the home. Beecher is in the hospital at St. Rose. He has bronchitis. The hospital is close by so it didn't take me long to get there. They gave him some meds and released him after running some tests. He had a high fever and was coughing a lot but they didn't feel a need to keep him overnight.

After this episode, I had to explain to the staff that Beecher has a DNR–Do Not Resuscitate. This was hard for me to do, but I had to instruct the caregivers to not call the ambulance every time he gets ill unless he is in pain. Since the hospital's job is to save patients, they will always do whatever possible to save him. This sounds uncaring, but it is just prolonging his life in a world of living where he has no quality of life.

~

May 30, Memorial Day

Went to visit Beecher to honor him. Took him a flag and some peanut butter cookies and a chocolate milkshake. Short stay. Very solemn today.

June 6

Diane called me and wanted me to bring some Vicks vapor rub for Beecher to put on at night. Took some to him and stopped at the store and also got some yogurt for him. The caregivers said he has been refusing to eat. Most of the time he won't open his mouth and when he does, he has a hard time swallowing. He ate the yogurt and he seemed to really like it and seemed happy too.

The caregivers said they noticed the decline. I talked with them and told them what to expect and that he wouldn't be getting any better. I think his time is coming soon. I think it might be time to call hospice pretty soon. I've been dreading this part of it.

I left and went to Sam's Club and bought him a whole box of yogurt and took it back to him. Tomorrow his sister Lola and family will be here. I hope that will cheer him up and they will have a nice visit with him. Amy went by to see him but he was in bed for the night so she didn't get to talk to him. She talked to Diane. She said Diane cried and said that she was very attached to him. Diane takes such good care of him. I hope Beecher can hang on for a while so we can visit with his sister.

Also, our 25th anniversary is coming up next week on June 15 and I would like him to still be here for that. I hope I'm not being selfish but I hope that he will be. Myra and one of the other caregivers said that sometimes he just starts crying. After all this time, I don't know if I'm ready for this. I'm trying so hard to let go but I really don't want to.

June 7

Beecher's sister Lola, Marc and Adele came to visit. Was so good to see them. Adele is now 14 and quite the artist. She is very shy and it took her awhile to warm up to Uncle Beech. She brought him one of her stuffed animals, a pelican. He never let go of it while we were there. Also, Amy came by. We got a few smiles out of Beecher and took some pictures. He ate some more yogurt and liked the watermelon strawberry Julius drink I bought him. At lease Beech is drinking more liquids. Diane said he has not been urinating much. Another sign of decline. We were there several hours and had a good visit. Lola said she was so happy they came now as she can see that it won't be much longer. Diane called me on the way home and said one of his meds was delivered today and it had melted due to the high heat we are having. Will go to the VA Pharmacy tomorrow to get it replaced.

∼

June 8

Got up early to go to VA to pick up the replacement med. Bad news! Got a call from the VA Pension Dept. They advised me that his pension would go down over $400 next month, due to the decrease in the cost of the group home which is $200 less than I was paying before. I asked them if they had received my latest expense statement and they said yes. Don't know how they figure such a lower amount. Probably won't be getting it much longer anyway because of his condition. Went to the VA and found out they no longer have a pharmacy at the clinic he goes to. Can only get scripts out at the VA hospital which is an hour's drive from my house each way.

Went to a luncheon with my daughter Michelle at the Brain Center called "Alive Inside." It was about how music impacts people with Dementia. It was excellent! Ran into my friends, Diane and John. John is in my watercolor class and Diane is a playwright and editor. Diane lost her mother to PSP, Progressive Supranuclear Palsy, several years ago.

Hope to someday have her help me edit this book if it ever comes to passing. Left the luncheon and drove out to the VA and picked up the medication. It was 116 degrees! Dropped off the meds to the group home. Beecher wasn't doing too well. Had a temp of 102. Wasn't eating much except yogurt. Talked to Francesca, the director and she agreed that he was declining. Gave me a number of a social worker to call at Nathan Adelson Hospice. She said they generally have to get the primary doctor to approve an assessment and they will come out to the home to do that. If approved, the hospice will stay at the home until Beecher passes. Just don't know who will pay for their service. We don't qualify for Medicaid and Beecher is not on Medicare health services, only hospitalization. When I got home, I called and left a message. Hope to hear something tomorrow.

Amy and Stephanie stopped by and took Beecher a watermelon smoothie. She said he drank most of it and also ate another yogurt and some dinner that was pureed. I guess he was feeling better but he still felt warm.

Ok, so going out again tonight to hear Amy and Stephanie sing at The Tuscany. Amy is doing a duet with Bucky Heard, who now performs with Bill Medley from the Righteous Brothers. They are going to sing the song called "Don't Know Much" by Linda Ronstadt (One of Beecher's and mine song). The night is a tribute to female singers, including Linda Ronstadt, Olivia Newton John, and Helen Reddy. Should be a good show. Lola and Marc will be there, too. It will be another late night for me, but of course I can't miss it. Going to video tape it so I can play it for Beecher tomorrow. Tomorrow will be a year since he was admitted to the first group home.

June 9

Today has been a year since Beecher went to the first group home. Can't believe another year has passed watching him decline. So hard to see him like this. Every stage is worse than the last one. Went to visit him and met Lola, Amy, Stephanie, Michelle & Frisco there. Beecher's fever is gone and he is eating a little better, but everything has to be pureed. He drank the watermelon Julius, I took him and he let me feed him pureed spaghetti. Yummy! NOT! But at least he is eating. Diane, the caregiver, said she has a hard time getting him out of the chair and into the wheelchair. His legs have no strength anymore. Takes two of them to do it and she used to be able to do by herself. He is having a harder time playing his iPad but he still attempts to try. I played the recorded video of the song Amy sang last night at the club. He watched it the whole time while Stephanie filmed both of us. It was so sweet, sentimental and emotional. I think he was trying to say something and he was tapping his fingers. We were all in tears.

Saturday, we are all going over to Michelle's for a BBQ. With Beecher's weakened condition, it would be too hard to take him. Sunday, Lola and I will go visit him again. And then again on Tuesday before she goes home. Wednesday the 15th is our 25th Anniversary. I'm going to make something special for Beecher to eat. Amy and Michelle will go over too. Something simple this year. Just want to spend some time with him again as I know it will probably be our last anniversary together.

Left several messages for the Social Worker at the VA in regards to Hospice. Should hear something on Monday. Our good friend Janon, a psychic, texted me after seeing the post on Facebook. Said she has been having a pressing feeling to come and visit him. We are going to try and hook up on Thursday at the home. Also, Belinda wants to see him too. Will be a busy week.

~

June 10

Got a letter from IRS today. They are auditing us for the year 2013! Can't believe it! Talk about bad timing! Just what I need. Called my CPA. Have to take all the receipts to her to copy so she can send them in ASAP. Only have 30 days. They call it a mail in audit. It sucks!

June 11

Nice BBQ at Michelle's house. Lola and family came and Amy too. Kids swam in pool. Took Beecher's albums to show Lola. She enjoyed seeing them and took pictures of some of the poems Beecher wrote. We're all going to visit Beech tomorrow. Amy got tickets to see the Righteous Brother's again. Another great evening! Bill Medley has a book out called "The Time of My Life." I bought a copy and left it in the restroom. Nobody turned it in even though it had been signed by Bill to me.

June 12

Visited Beech. Still eating about the same. Lola and family came. Beech fist bumped his nephew, Sammy. That was something different for him. One of his other sisters, Cricket, called. We put the phone to Beecher's ear so she could talk to him and he could listen to her. You could tell by the look on his face that he knew who it was. Nice visit. Got a few smiles from him. He even looked at me for about 20 seconds. Fed him some baked beans I made. He seemed to like them, and they are soft and easy to eat.

June 13

Spent the day with my girlfriends from Las Vegas High School. Went to the Neon Museum and then had lunch at Jerry's Nugget afterwards. It was good to have a down day. Spending time with friends always seems to lighten my load.

June 14

A very sad bittersweet day. Lola and family had to leave to go back home. They came to visit him for the last time. I cried so hard for her. I know it will be the last time she will see her brother. At least she got to visit with him a lot while they were here.

June 15

Our 25th anniversary! What a special day! Took some lobster and baked potatoes to Beecher along with a card and a poem that I wrote him. Amy, Michelle, Andrea, Stephanie, Justin and Bethany came. Also, Amy's friend Rick Duarte came to sing and play the guitar. Amy and Stephanie sang along as well. The music was awesome and they were all the songs Beecher and I love so dearly. I played a song for Beecher that I had recorded by Carole King called "Now and Forever" and read the card and the poem that I had written for him. We ate Eggplant Parmesan that Stephanie made, had an awesome cake, a lot of laughter and a lot of tears that made for a very special memorable day. The music seemed to help Beech come alive. We saw him tapping him fingers at times and also opening his eyes when he recognized a song that he loved. I owe a ton of thanks to my daughters and the rest of my family and friends for sharing this special day with us. I am so blessed to have them all in my life!

June 16

Rested pretty much today. I'm exhausted! Been a long week. Made one trip out to visit Beech for a few minutes. He was having trouble with his iPad. Got it fixed and then came right home.

June 19

Father's Day-swimming and dinner at my brother Ricky's house then off to visit Beech.

~

June 20

Tax appointment for 2013 audit. UGH!

~

June 22

Appointment for Beecher with his new primary doctor at the VA, Dr. Stevens. Had a rough time getting Beecher out of my car and back into the car. Weight and blood pressure are down some more. 169 lbs. and 101/67. Visit went well and this new doctor is a really nice lady. She is actually a nurse practitioner. Very compassionate. I liked her a lot. I started crying at one point and she empathized with me. Beecher heard me crying and he looked up in a caring way and she walked over to him and patted him on the shoulder. She told him it was OK and that I was just worried about him. She even helped me get him from the wheelchair into the car. She will try to help me get Hospice for him. I have to coordinate with Dr. Léger at the Brain Center if he thinks he is ready for it and will send a certified letter to Dr. Stevens. When I got Beecher back to the home, I fed him his lunch and ice cream and he ate everything. When I left, he looked up at me and I blew him a kiss and he tried blowing one back to me. I was crying by the time I got to the car. Went back at three to visit him with Amy and Michelle to celebrate a late Father's Day. Michelle made some bread pudding and brought it to him. Nice visit with him. Amy brought her iPad with videos from the Air Supply concert she went to and gave him an Air Supply t-shirt. He watched all the videos and ate the bread pudding. You could tell he loved it all.

~

June 23

I went to see Beecher and I brought him a chocolate milkshake and he could hardly let go of it. I think he's missed it! Also, I took his iPod and his headset to him and he had it on almost the whole time except for when he was watching Amy sing "Me and Bobby McGee." He had his eyes open almost all the time that I was there! I clipped his toenails and his fingernails and I know he liked that. I fed him his lunch and he ate everything. Good day with him! I pushed the iPad down in his chair on his left side so hopefully he won't mess around with it. He keeps messing with it and causes it to lock up. He was doing good with his Angry Birds today also. Also told him I loved him and he looked at me and mouthed the words back!

~

June 24

Visit with Dr. Léger today. At this time, Francesca takes him to the appointment and I meet her there. It is getting harder for me to transport him by myself due to his falls. Dr. Léger estimated maybe six months prognosis. He saw the decline. Body very stiff. He rated Beech at a level 7(d) on the FAST track criteria for hospice and said he would send a letter to his primary. He agreed with me as to keeping him at the home and not sending him to a skilled nursing home. Because he has a terminal degenerative disease, they would prolong his life instead of letting it take its course. He also said the use of antibiotics would prolong it and it would be my decision on the use of them. At one point I got emotional and Beech opened his eyes and looked up at me. Dr Léger told him I was worried about him and I assured him I was ok. Dr Léger said he still has a sensitivity to my feelings. We will see him again in three months. Per doctor's notes: There is a steady progression of the disease over the last many months. There is complete dependence on assist of two people to transfers. Early difficulties sitting up without assistance. Increased difficulty with swallowing and choking. Incontinence in both bowel and bladder. Bed sores have become more difficult to manage. "His prognosis and depending on the aggressiveness of treatment of complications (pneumonia and UTI , that his prognosis is less than six months.)" He added ENSURE to his medications. Also, he no longer tries to get up on his own so he is relatively safe. His weight is now 170 lbs. He recommended he would greatly benefit from Hospice Care.

*Note: Medicare's dementia criteria for eligibility for Hospice are:

Life expectancy is six months or less

The person is unable to ambulate, bathe, or dress independently

Urinary or fecal incontinence

No consistently meaningful verbal communication – speech limited to six or fewer words

One of more of the following has occurred in the past year:

Aspiration pneumonia, kidney/upper urinary-tract infection, septicemia, recurring fever after antibiotics, ulcers (pressure sores) multiple stage 3-4, unexplained weight loss of 10% or more in the past six months and blood levels of albumin concentration that measure less than 25mg. which is generally associated with malnourishment.

Getting hospice care for FTD patients is sometimes challenging as the criteria was originally based on the progression of Alzheimer's disease, (AD). People with FTD are different because FTD impacts different areas of the brain and are generally younger. Memory impairment may not be severe as AD, but the risk for falls is significantly higher. These differences from AD may mistakenly lead clinicians unfamiliar with FTD to believe that patients with FTD are not at the end-of-life because they still look pretty good.

There is a critical need to raise awareness to the signs and symptoms that may indicate the end of life in persons with FTD.

I believe Beecher qualifies for all of the above.

Note: Death from Late–Stage Dementia. Many individuals with late-stage dementia die of a medical complication such as pneumonia or another infection. However, dementia itself is fatal. General wasting, malnutrition and dehydration are genuine risks when an individual with dementia can no longer eat safely and or move independently.

~

July 5

Took Beecher a doughnut. Custard filled with chocolate icing. His favorite! I asked him if he liked it to give me a thumbs-up which he did. Then I asked him if he loves me to give me a thumbs-up and he did. Then I asked him if he really, really loves me to give me two thumbs-up and he gave me two thumbs-up! It's amazing how he still follows some commands and it lets me know he is still in there somewhere. God, I love days like this when he is so responsive. It really saddens me that he can't be like this all the time. I miss the person he used to be, but I'll settle for any little glimpse of him that I can get. I know in my heart that his time is short and I may not get many more of these days. I realize it's the little things that count!

~

July 8

Thirty-two years ago, today my dear Mother passed away. It's also my oldest granddaughter Leah's wedding day and Michelle's and Cole's Anniversary! I just got a call from the VA and they have approved Hospice care for Beecher. They will pay for everything. Nathan Adelson will be contacting me to set up an appointment to assess him. Finally got this approved! I know Mom is watching out over us. As I am writing this, Nathan Adelson just called me to set up an appointment for the assessment. We set it up for Monday morning the 11th and guess what the name of the nurse is? Nurse Amy! My Mother's really got it covered!

Leah's and Craig's wedding day! What a beautiful wedding it was at the Paiute Golf Resort. Leah sang a song to her husband and it was absolutely beautiful. Then Amy got up and sang the song "Kiss Me." It was wonderful seeing all three of my granddaughters and her family. Beecher would have loved the wedding. Wish he could have gone.

July 9

Woke up this morning sick. Maybe something I ate. I had promised Michelle, I would help her out with the craft show today. She wasn't feeling good either but we did the show and got through it and it was a good day for her money wise. Ate half of a sandwich to get something in my stomach. Then went to meet up with my Granddaughters so they could visit Beecher before they head back home to Utah. Did I tell you my granddaughter Suzie is pregnant and she is due in November? She mentioned she might name her baby boy Beech or maybe for his middle name. I think she was serious. She said she liked the name. Don't want to put any pressure on her but I think she really wants to. I know Beech would love that as he always used to say to women that were pregnant (Beecher's a good name). Anyway, said my goodbyes and came home feeling nauseated again so I took some Alka-Seltzer and went to bed. Spent half the night on the toilet. Hope I feel better tomorrow.

July 11

Met with Nathan Adelson Hospice Nurse Administrator, Kristie and she approved Beech for hospice. They have ordered a hospital bed, gel pad, wheelchair, shower chair, porta potty for his room and all the supplies that he needs. They will be in charge of the medications through VA and VA will pay all the costs. The nurse administrator was wonderful and she covered everything including trying to get him visits seven days a week but at least five days if not. She talked to Beecher and told him who she was. I explained to Beecher so he understood and told him to squeeze my hand if the situation was OK with him. He squeezed my hand slightly which made me feel good. I made sure he knew he was not leaving the home he's in but he would be staying there and the hospice would visit him there. He seemed to be OK with everything. I was there almost four hours while Kristie was getting everything taken care of. When I left, Kristie hugged me several times and told me that I was doing a good job taking care of him and that I was a good advocate for him. This made me cry. She said the social worker would be getting in touch with me for any questions I had in regards to his funeral and also if I needed spiritual support. I said yes that would be nice.

~

July 12

Went to visit Beech for a short time to take his iPod back to him with a new cord so he could listen to music. Lucy, the new nurse that will be taking care of Beech was there. The hospice had already sent the bed and other supplies and already had them set up. Lucy explained to me that she would be coming three days a week which is a little different than what I was told but we will get to the bottom of that she said.

After I left, I stopped at Walmart to do some shopping and Chaplain Dan from Hospice called me. I talked to him briefly and he asked me if I would like him to visit Beecher. I said yes, I think that would be nice. It's been an emotional couple of days knowing that his life is soon to be over. I am very sad about this and having a hard time letting go but I know when the time comes it will be better for him as well as for me and my family.

Today I signed the patient DNR request form with Nathan Adelson Hospice, consenting to only palliative care to maintain comfort. The DNR means that if his heart stops beating or he stops breathing, no medical procedures to start breathing or heart function will be instituted. This was Beecher 's request on his Living Will which he signed in 2006. I also signed a form stating I had elected to use the Hospice Medicare VA Benefit with Nathan Adelson Hospice concerning payments and other consent forms for services from Nathan Adelson. I think I am in a daze that it has finally come to this. It feels like I am giving up but I know that taking care of someone with a serious illness, especially at home, without hospice is like trying to have surgery without anesthesia. As much as I would have liked to bring him home to die (to keep with my commitment to never put him in a home), I had to make that decision last year when I realized I could not care for him any longer at home. As much as I wanted to believe I could do it, it was just no longer feasible and he did not contest it anyway. So, I feel I made the best decision but it still hurts my heart. Sometimes those promises you make on your wedding day are just no longer feasible and are really the best thing for both of you.

Now that I've been through this process, I realize that hospice is designed to support more personal aspects of this life stage, reflecting on one's legacy and life meaning and focusing on relationships in a deeper and more intentional way, achieving a sense of closure and realizing any end-of-life goals and getting financial affairs in order. This brought me and my daughters closer than I had ever imagined and we were already close. Watching someone die but living with them until the end of life can't help but bring you closer and bring closure to someone you love with all your heart. These last few years my husband has had no quality of life except what we were able to offer him, celebrating his birthdays, our anniversaries, the holidays and painting which brought him so much joy. I now have so many good memories and a book of his paintings to cherish a lifetime. Hospice is bringing back some of that quality of life as well by making sure Beecher doesn't suffer any more than he needs to, and for us to know that his suffering is being managed.

~

July 13

Took the day off from all this and went with my next-door neighbor Kathy to go to the new IKEA store. Had a nice day and ate lunch there and didn't get home until after four o'clock. Was a nice break for me.

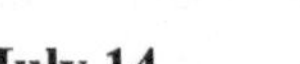

July 14

Short visit with Beech to take him some Twinkies and a Slurpee which he loved. Suzie's boyfriend, Aaron asked me the other day if he thought that Beech and I would approve of him asking Suzie, my granddaughter to marry him. Aaron is the father of her baby. I took a video asking Beecher if he would approve and he gave me a thumbs-up and a fist bump which is definitely a yes! I sent the video of Beecher to Aaron and he was very happy! Also, Bridgett, the social worker, from hospice called me this morning and asked me some questions. I will follow up with her tomorrow. They did approve to visit him five days a week Monday through Friday and also included two nurses to help him shower. Got another call from a nurse named Kim from hospice in regards to his meds. I will follow up tomorrow also. This is all becoming so surreal.

July 15

Got a call today from Beecher's nephew Tyler. Good news and bad news. Tyler's wife Shawna is expecting a baby girl in December. Also, his brother Terry and his wife Brittany are expecting a baby in December. He's going to try to get up to visit Beecher pretty soon. Bad news is their mother Kitty just found out she has rectal cancer stage four. She lives up in Reno. So sad to hear that. Visited Beecher for about an hour and then went by to check on Amy's cat Phoebe, (my Grand Kitty), while Amy is in Alaska for a few days. Beecher was in a quiet mood but he ate all of his lunch and ice cream. Another long hot day, 116!

As of this date, Beecher is on the following medications:

- Quetiapine (Seroquel) for sleep and an antidepressant -100mg, 1 tab at night

- Omeprazole for acid reflux – 20mg – 1 tablet before meal in the AM
- Lisinopril for blood pressure – 10 mg- 1 tab in the AM
- Senna syrup 8.8 mg. 3 times a day for constipation prevention
- Lexapro – 10 mg – 1 tab in AM as an antidepressant
- Tylenol – 325 mg - 1 tab 2 times a day as needed for pain
- Morphine Sulfate Concentrate –by mouth 20 mg/Ml 5 mg every hour
- Lactulose by mouth 20 GM/30Ml daily if no BM for 3 days
- Trazodone HCI by mouth – 100 mg 3 tabs (300mg) every evening at bedtime
- Trazodone HCI by mouth – 100 mg 2 tabs (200mg) every AM
- Hydroxyzine Pamoate by moth 25mg – 1 cap 2 times a day as needed at PM for anxiety

July 16

My sister Linda is coming to town to stay for a week. She is staying at my brother Ricky's until Monday morning and then I'll go pick her up.

July 18

Picked up Linda from Ricky's house and we drove out to Lake Las Vegas. We met my sister Patti out there and her niece Sarah and her boyfriend Jason. Patti drove us up to Mount Charleston which was much cooler than it is here in Vegas. Had a nice time and walked around a little bit. We went to the visitor center and bought some puzzles for my nephews since I missed all three of their birthdays this year. Drove back to Lake Las Vegas and the three of us went to dinner at Luna Rosa, our favorite Italian restaurant. Had a great time. Linda had rented a room for all three of us to stay the night but Patti decided not to stay.

∽

July 19

Checked out of our room and drove into Vegas to have lunch with Patti's niece Sarah at Mimi's café. Great crepes! Said goodbye to Sarah and her boyfriend and the three of us girls went to the movies to see Ghostbusters at Green Valley Ranch. Came back to my house after stopping at Whole Foods where we bought some lobster dinners for us.

∽

July 20

Beecher had a doctor's appointment at the VA so Linda and I met him and the director there. First time my sister Linda has seen him since last April when she was here visiting. Appointment went well with the mental health provider and it was decided Beecher no longer needed to come because the Hospice is now handling all of his medication.

We went to the movies with Patti again. Movie called "Mike and Dave Needs Wedding Dates." It was hilarious. I needed a good laugh or two.

∽

July 21

Linda and I hung around the house for a while then went to work out at the Solera clubhouse. In the evening, we went to see a play out at Spring Mountain Ranch called "Memphis." Amy went with us and we had a great time. It was much cooler in the mountains. We took some salads and wine and just chilled out. Boy, I sure needed that too.

∽

July 22

Linda and I took a walk around the block and then went to visit Beecher. Had a real nice visit with him as he was very engaged with Linda and I. She showed him some videos of her grandkids in the jacuzzi and he really liked that. One of the best visits I've had with him in a while and very happy that he was so engaged.

Linda got to see him as the child that he is now. After that just hung around the house until it was time to go meet Ricky and Chris at the Palazzo to see a musical called "Baz." Great show and fun being out with my sister and my brother!

July 23

Went to see Amy perform at Pancho's Mexican restaurant with her friend Rick Duarte. Another great night and late night. Wow three nights in a row. I'm getting too old for this. It sure was fun though! Michelle and Cole also came down to watch Amy including Cole's son, Cam who is visiting here from Arizona and their little boy Lucas also came.

July 24

Sad day. Linda had to go home. I sure enjoyed visiting with her and we got to do a lot of things and she got to see a lot of family and especially Beecher. It was a great having her here and getting to spend so much time with her. I really needed a nice week of respite. It was a lot of fun and a lot of laughs. I miss her already and she's only been gone a half-day.

August 4

Met with caseworker Melinda. She is a very nice lady. Said Beecher's vital signs were good 120/80. Beecher has a bad yeast infection on his bottom surrounding his bedsore. The Hospice ordered meds to clear it up. Should be almost gone within the week. He doesn't seem to be in any pain. Still feel bad for him--going through so much--so sad.

~

August 7

Today's visit with Beecher went well. He continues to play with the Turtle toy I gave him. He likes the music, especially the song "Alueta" which he plays over and over. He looked up at me a few times and stared at me for a minute or so. He was also listening to his iPod on the radio I brought over. When the song "Tie a Yellow Ribbon Round the Old Oak Tree" by Tony Orlando came on, I started singing along to it. When it got to the part, "Do You Still Want me?' I asked him to give me a thumbs-up and he did and he did it twice! It's amazing how he still responds. The Hospice sent him a Certificate thanking him for his service in the military. It had his name on it. When I showed it to him, he grabbed on to the end of the paper to look at it. I asked him to point to his name and he pointed right to it! There is still so much of him in there, it's unbelievable! Diane said his yeast infection is clearing up but he is eating less food.

~

August 10

Had a very good visit with Beecher today. I surprised him with a watercolor book that I had made through Shutterfly. It was a book with pictures of all the paintings he had painted since 2013. His eyes opened so big when he saw it and he turned each page and looked at each picture and pointed to some of them when I named the picture. I think he was really proud of it.

I called Diane into the other room to talk to her about Beecher's brain donation and said that I would bring her a piece of paper with the phone number of someone she would have to call at the time of Beecher's death. She started crying and said that it was very hard for her because she is very fond of Beecher. She is a wonderful caregiver and I know she will miss him. Afterwards she went outside for a few minutes and then came back in and sat next to him in his chair. I left feeling very sad for her and for Beecher and myself. Some days it is just so hard to see him like he is, but on the other hand, I feel so blessed for all the memories he has made for me. Making his book will give me something more to remember him by as I am very proud of all the paintings he has done.

I received a message from Dr. Léger that Cleveland Clinic has secured funding that will allow for brain donation, whenever that time comes. He also mentioned that they would need a blood sample while Beecher is still alive for research purposes and that someone would be contacting me and paperwork would be needed. He asked me if I would mind speaking to a reporter for the Review Journal. He said the reporter had been in his office today to report on their telemedicine. She had asked about Beecher's big horn sheep watercolor which is in Dr. Léger's office. Beecher had given it to the doctor some time ago. The reporter said the RJ would be very interested in featuring Beecher's story and if I was interested, Dr. Léger would reach out to them and ask them to call me. Of course, I said yes.

~

August 11

Beecher had an appointment at the VA today with his primary doctor but I cancelled it. It is too hard to transport him and besides he is on Hospice and they know what to do. Today I signed the Tissue Donation Advanced Medical Directive to remove and retain Beecher's brain and tissue for research and educational uses only. Common information about Brain

Donation is as follows: All costs involved in brain donations, including transportation of the brain to Cleveland Clinic in Ohio will be paid by the Brain Center. A person can still have an open casket at a funeral as the process of removing the brain is done is such a way that allows an open casket. In cases of cremations, you can be cremated by the funeral home of your choice. Donated tissue is kept in a Cleveland Clinic facility for scientific study, and storage. Researchers from across the country may request tissue samples to conduct approved research. Specimens and data will be connected to a unique ID number so that no researcher will be able to identify the person. In Beecher's case I would have to find a mortuary that could do the brain removal where a certified technician could come and remove Beecher's brain within 24 hours after death. His body would be sent to the facility (mortuary) where his brain is to be removed. In Las Vegas, Desert Memorial was the only one that has a prep room for pathology personnel to come and remove his brain. As time is of the essence, it has to be a local pathologist and the prep room must be available seven days a week. The fee is $250 for use of the room and available from nine to five daily and will be paid for by the Brain Center. Desert Memorial will also do the cremation after his brain is removed. The most important aspect is to notify all caregivers, hospice and family that Beecher's brain is being donated and what needs to happen immediately upon his death especially in the event that I am not near at the time of death. A Tissue Donation Intent Card must be in my possession (wallet) at all times and a copy must be kept in the care facility in Beecher's medical record chart. All persons must understand the severity of making the call to the Cleveland Clinic Foundation upon death and state: "My loved one has passed away and is a Center for Brain Health tissue donor. I was told that I should call immediately so that my loved one's body can be transported for tissue removal and ask them to please page the technician as soon as possible" The phone number for the Foundation is located on the Tissue Donation Card which should be posted nearby, preferably in his room. The Intent card should have at least three contact numbers of family in case no one is there at the time of death. The Foundation operator will contact the Tissue Donation Team and ambulance transportation arrangements will be made. His body will then be transported for tissue removal and then released to the funeral home of choice. Once the Foundation receives his brain, they will notify me and I should receive the pathology report in approximately three to four months. The report will include DNA info and any other causes of death, like stroke, and may include any genetic info.

~

August 12

A very nice day today. I went to lunch with some of my friends from high school. I took the watercolor book I had made for Beecher and shared it with them. They really liked it. Then I went to visit Beecher and I took his watercolor book with me again so he could look at it. It was such a blessed beautiful day as two of the ladies that are residents there came over to look at his book with him. One of the ladies, named Miriam, said that he always waves to her when she is sitting at the table having her meals. She then grabbed his hand and told him he was a great artist. She also stroked his head and said that she likes to do that because she knows that he likes that. I asked Beech if he liked his book to give me a thumbs-up which he did. He actually gave me two thumbs-up. One of the other residents, named Yum, was also standing there looking at the watercolor book and she kept giving Beech a thumbs-up. It is so nice to see that the residents love and respect each other and that it is really a truly loving care facility. I am so blessed and fortunate that he is at a home in which he is loved not only by the caregivers but by the other residents as well. They seem to watch out for each other and it is evident that they really care about Beecher. That just fills my heart with so much love.

After that, one of the other residents named Martha, who is wheel-chair-bound, is almost blind and very heavyset but is such a beautiful soul, asked if she could see the book. She heard us talking about his book and she wanted to know if she could see it. I took it over to her and she said that she could see up close and see colors. I turned all the pages for her and she loved what she saw, at least, what she could see. She said that it was very nice of me to make the book for him. After she looked at the book she asked if she could give me a hug. She said she had just had a shower and I said it would be OK anyway. I leaned down and hugged her and let her hug me. It was a special moment. There are truly so many amazing human beings in this world that we don't always think about just because they are in a home. I thank God for each and every one of them including the caregivers who have so much love. I feel so surrounded by love when I walk into the room to see my husband and to share things with the other residents. These memories I will always carry close to my heart. It was truly a beautiful wonderful day. Thank you, God for allowing these people into my life. I wouldn't be able to carry this burden if it wasn't for them and my family and my friends. Just before I left, Rita, one of the caregivers, gave me some of her homemade eggrolls! She knows how much I love them. She is so sweet as are all of them at the home. I am so blessed!

August 15

Visited Beecher today. He was pretty quiet but he ate most of his food, especially the ice cream. I showed him his book again and he looked through about half of it and then he closed his eyes. He seemed very distant today and not looking at me much. Although he did give a thumbs-up to Dan, the Chaplain, when Dan told him it was a very nice book that I made for him. Beecher always seems to follow me with his eyes when I'm talking to the other residents but sometimes when I'm sitting by him, he won't look at me. I also found out today that Myra is no longer there and that she had moved back to the Philippines. I was sad to hear that as she was my other favorite caregiver.

Got the call from the reporter, Pash from the RJ, who asked to do a story on Beecher and his artwork. I have a telephone interview with her on Wednesday. The story will focus on Beecher, his passion for artwork, experience at the Brain Center and his diagnosis. The reporter really loved Beecher's artwork and wants to include some of his pictures in the article. I'm anxious to see the article when it comes out. And of course, I will take a copy to Beecher. Also, a lady from the Cleveland Clinic called me in regards to the bio bank which is blood work they take to do a study for research. They are sending me some forms to go over and then I have to call them to get Beech in the program. There is no cost for this blood draw. The research study is designed to answer specific questions about new ways to detect, diagnose, treat and prevent disease. I felt it was necessary to participate as you never know when the study might help someone else, although no report would be made available to me.

August 16

I got the consent form for the blood draw. The lady that contacted me said they would send out the supplies to TLC to do the blood draw. The nurse from Hospice can do the draw. They may draw up to one half cup of blood from his vein. The blood sample will be used for obtaining genetic material (DNA) and extracting plasma or serum to measure certain proteins or other substances found in the blood. A portion of the blood may be sent to Cleveland Clinic laboratory for testing, (i.e., complete blood count).

Once it's completed, it will be determined by the Principal Investigator. The results will be placed in Beecher's medical record. If DNA is unable to be collected via blood draw, a saliva sample may be used to obtain DNA. As far as the research study, Beecher was not available to do any of their further testing, i.e., cognitive testing, which would have included a short test of his memory, because of his decline and inability to speak. If a researcher identifies a gene in his DNA that is known to cause a certain disease or condition, I have the option to be notified that a genetic change has been found and I can be referred for further confirmatory genetic testing regarding further testing.

August 17

Spoke to the RJ reporter today. Very good interview, I think. They want five or six pictures of his to put in the article which I sent to them. Also, they want a photographer to come out and take a picture of Beecher and I and also to meet us. I expressed that what I wanted out of the article was to bring awareness of the disease to help other people get a quicker diagnosis. I told her Beecher's brain is being donated for research so it will help find a cure and what causes FTD. I am meeting with them next Tuesday at the home.

Met Michelle at the home and we visited Beecher and then went to lunch. Had a nice visit with her and had a great talk. This is just hard for everybody. I wish I could take away the pain that they all feel. Everyone loves him so much and he made such a great impact in their lives.

August 18

Made some calls to some mortuaries today in regards to brain donation and cremation. Talked to several of them and made the decision on Desert Memorial because they can do the brain donation there as well as the cremation. Called hospice and told them of my decision for Desert Memorial. Glad to have that done as I was putting it off and it needed to be done. Tomorrow, I need to get a hold of Social Security and find out what my total Social Security will be after Beecher is gone. So much to do, even when I think I've got everything handled, there's always something else. I will be glad when all of this is over so I can just relax and not think about this horrible disease and how it's affected me and my family's life. I know I am going to miss him but I am so ready for this part to be over and be past it. I know why they call this disease "The Long Goodbye."

August 19

Nice visit with Beecher today. Took him a chocolate milkshake. He kept his eyes closed most of the time while he drank it. I fed him his lunch, puréed spaghetti again. How boring. He ate it but didn't seem too thrilled about it. Except for the ice cream of course. I took one of our albums from 2007; we did several cruises that year. Beech turned some of the pages and looked at the pictures but then closed his eyes about halfway through. At one point while he had his eyes open and looking at me, I told him I loved him and I asked him to give me a smile and he gave me almost a half a smile. That seems to be the best that he can do these days. He seems to decline more and more each week, with less interaction and fewer thumbs-up. It's so sad to watch. Called Social Security and found out that since I'm over 66, I will get Beecher's full Disability amount. All I have to do is call them. There will be no interruption in payments. I can also call S.S. and get Death Benefits of $250. No need to go down to S.S. I can do everything over the phone. That is such a relief. Have to remind myself now to cancel his A & A (VA Pension) as well when this is over.

~

August 23

I met with the photographer and reporter from the RJ (Review Journal) and the coordinator from Cleveland Clinic at TLC. It went very well. They did a video of me and Beecher and also took pictures. They were there for almost two hours. The article will be printed in the RJ and also a video on YouTube. I didn't know about the video until today. But I think it will be great and it is a good way of getting out our story about this dreadful disease and about Beecher's passion for painting. Beecher was responsive at different times. He even smiled when I talked about him looking like Jesse Ventura the wrestler whom he was told he looked like at one point in his life. The photographer Jeff and Pash the reporter were wonderful, as well as MacKenzie the coordinator from Cleveland

Clinic. We shared a lot of stories about Beecher and the person he was and how the disease has affected him in so many ways. After they left, I sat with Beecher for a while and held his hand and I asked him several times to squeeze my hand. He did four different times. That's better than nothing since he can't do the "I love you" sign in sign language anymore. At least I know he's still in there somewhere. It was a good day!

August 24

Met Melinda the case manager for Hospice at TLC. B/P 110/80. The caregivers transferred him into his room. His yeast infection has not cleared up. She now thinks it may be something else. She decided to cover it this time. If it gets worse, then it is a yeast infection and they will have to do something different. He was very quiet today and had his eyes closed almost all the time I was there. Melinda and the caregivers agreed that soon he would be bedridden as they are having a hard time transferring him from the wheelchair or the recliner into his bed. His body has become so stiff it is hard to get him moved. He keeps crossing his right leg over his left leg even when he stands up to walk so they don't want to make him walk anymore. They put him right into the wheelchair to get him to the bathroom and to bed. His right foot seems to be turned in and maybe that's why he crosses it. I noticed a red spot on his left ankle. Melinda checked it and said, yes, he was getting another bedsore. She put a patch over it. He seems so out of it today almost like he is semi-conscious. It just broke my heart to see him like this. I can't stand this much longer. I just feel so bad for him. Got a message from MacKenzie from the RJ and she said they had interviewed Dr. Léger last Friday. Dr. Léger let them know that the FTD awareness week is actually the last week of September. They are going to try to go out with the article then, but MacKenzie will let me know.

August 26

Frances went with me to visit Beech. I gave her a copy of the Watercolor book I made him. She loved it. We had a nice visit with Beecher. He squeezed my hand and also Frances's hand several times. At one point he stared into my eyes for several minutes and seemed to be listening to me as I told him how much I loved him. I told him I appreciated him for always taking care of me and that's why I'm taking care of him now. I hadn't seen that look in his eyes in quite a while and he seemed to adore me at that moment. It was wonderful. I will always cherish that feeling that I had with him today.

August 28

Nice visit with Beech today. Clipped his fingernails and fed him his dinner. Rita made me some eggrolls and some rice so I ate it while I fed him. He kept looking over at the chili sauce so I put it on some of his purée meatloaves and potato. He seemed to like it. One of the resident's named Dan is in the hospital. Don't know what's wrong with him but I hope he's ok. I showed Beecher some of the videos from Amy singing at Pancho's last night and he seemed to like that.

August 30

I talked to Melinda the case manager from hospice today. She said the yeast infection on his bottom is not actually a yeast infection but she believes it is just a scar from the yeast infection that he had. She also said he has a tender spot on his right ankle and he pulls away when it is touched. She says he has another bed sore on his bottom just starting. Melinda told me the caregivers say that he seems to be in pain when he gets up every morning. I think they are going to start giving him morphine. It breaks my heart. I'm feeling more and more like the end is near and I hate this part.

~

August 31

Went to visit Beecher, and Michelle met me there. Beecher wasn't being very responsive today; however, he did squeeze my hand and Michelle's hand. His left ankle on the inside was bandaged today instead of the outside. Also, his right foot was turned in more and I could see an indentation where it is evidently sore. Diane gave him some morphine and said she is giving it to him twice a day. I took him some tapioca pudding and he seemed to enjoy that. I left three more for them to feed him. I think he is declining very fast now and probably will be bedridden soon. Michelle and I left and went to lunch at the Bonefish Grill. We had a good time and had lots to talk about. Hopefully, in two weeks, Amy can start meeting us for lunch also on every other Wednesday.

~

September 1

I had a relaxing day or at least part of it. Went to watercolor class and almost finished the picture of Michelle's dog Frisco, (my Grand Puppy). Can't wait to finish it and give it to her. Painting always calms me down and de-stresses me. Went to the dentist and had my front tooth filled. Glad to have that done. But not the $200 or so that it cost me. Oh well. Always something. Got a call from Amy. She got accepted into a new band called WolfCreek. She will be the only female in the band and they are very popular here in Las Vegas so it's a very good move for her and great for her music career. They will be performing at the T-Mobile arena in Las Vegas on September 10. I'm so excited for her! I talked to a friend of mine today and she told me to check with Touro University here in Las Vegas as they do organ donors and burial and everything at no charge. I will call them tomorrow just to get information even though I have already made my decision.

September 4

I had a brief visit with Beecher. The caregivers had him on the toilet when I got there. I saw that his right knee was bandaged with an ace bandage. I asked Diane about it and she said that it was kind of red and green. She unwrapped it to show me and it just looks like the vein on his knee was sticking out some. His right foot is still turning in more. That is probably what is causing his pain as his body is getting so stiff especially on that side. It took Diane, Rita and me to get Beecher off the toilet and into the wheelchair as it is hard for him to stand. We got Beecher back into the living room. Diane is giving him his morphine in a syringe now so that he won't waste too much. I took him a Starbucks frappe and he drank some of that. I didn't stay very long as I had to get home and fix my toilet. Beecher looked so sad today and I think he must just be as tired of this disease as I am.

When I got home, I got a call from my friend in California named Roz. She was crying and needed somebody to talk to as her husband is going through some issues and she feels like she has lost her husband as well. We had a good talk and decided we will keep in touch. She will be quitting her job in California and moving into her house in Arizona in December to take care of her husband who is in rehab right now. She stated to me that he is no longer the man she married. Many of his issues are unrelated to Beecher's but the doctor did say that he has a form of dementia. Her husband is 57. She feels much the same way that I do about the changes in her husband and how the plans they had in their old age are never going to happen. I feel for her as I know what she is going through. It is so difficult. I hope I can be there for her as much as she needs me. I pray for her and that she gets through this like I know I will and that we both will have a life again. Beecher and my golden years are gone and any hopes for our future together.

I wrote my response letter to the IRS and mailed it to them regarding the audit. I'll keep my fingers crossed that they allow the deductions, especially the unreimbursed expenses.

~

September 10

The new band WolfCreek that Amy just joined performed at the outside stage for the opening party for George Straight at the T-Mobile Arena. I went to watch her perform. I think country music is her genre! It was great but it was very hot being that it was outdoors! Afterwards she and the band got to see George Straight! I'm so jealous!

~

September 12

Great visit with Beecher today. My friend Belinda went with me. Beecher was quite attentive today. I showed him a video of Amy singing with the WolfCreek band at the T-Mobile Arena.

When it was over, I told him to clap if he liked it and he tried putting his two hands together. I was able to get a picture of him doing that. It was so sweet.

When Belinda and I got ready to leave I leaned over and kissed Beecher goodbye. Belinda told Beecher she would give him a kiss too but he had food on his mouth. I had just finished feeding him. He had a napkin in his hand so he tried to wipe his lips off so she could kiss him. It was pretty funny.

It's so weird sometimes how much he understands. She didn't kiss him on the lips but she did kiss him on the cheek and he seemed to like that. He also squeezed both of our hands before we left. So, I know he knew who we were and that he is feeling the love.

~

September 14

Met Melinda at the Home and visited Beech today. There is a new case manager starting next week name Jerri. The caregivers took Beecher in the bedroom so they could look at his bed sores. The one on his bottom is getting bigger and he's starting to get another one in the same area. There's also one on the back of his knee on his right leg and he still has one on his left ankle. Just hate seeing him like this. It is so sad; it just breaks my heart. After the case manager checked him over, Diane went ahead and put Beecher down for a nap so they wouldn't have to take him back out into the other room. She said they would get him up again at three before dinner. I had taken him a chocolate milkshake but he only got a sip of it before they took him into the bedroom. So, I put it in the refrigerator so he could have it later. I didn't get to visit him very much. I did walk into the bedroom to check on him before I left and when I walked in, he had his eyes open. I went over and kissed him and said goodbye and he closed his eyes. Poor guy. I don't even know if he is aware of what's going on. But to see his body deteriorating week after week and getting so frail and so thin, it just doesn't seem fair that he has to go through this.

~

September 17

Beecher's other friend Gary Rinebarger and his girlfriend Maggie came up to visit Beech from Arizona. Beecher was quite surprised to see him and his eyes opened up so big his forehead wrinkled. We knew immediately that he had recognized Gary. Gary grabbed Beecher's hand and held onto it for a long time. Beecher's hands were shaking so much today that he just held onto Gary's hand. It was a very nice visit. We didn't stay long because it was late in the afternoon and they were getting ready to put him to bed. I did notice that Beecher has an ace bandage on both of his legs now which means he is getting more bedsores. Afterwards, Gary, Maggie and I went and had some Thai food and then walked down

Fremont Street. Maggie had never been to Fremont Street. Had a real nice time but got to bed late. I'm sure I'll be very tired tomorrow.

September 18

Got up late but Gary, Maggie and I went to visit Beech before they headed back home to Arizona. It was a very emotional day. We stopped to get him a milkshake and some ice cream and Beecher really enjoyed all that. After he ate, we kept teasing him because he kept looking at Maggie and Gary kept saying, isn't she hot? She's a hot chick huh? You could almost see him smile. But instead, he closed one eye like he was winking at her. He did it twice. I was so surprised because he completely closed one eye. It was quite funny! Also, while I was there, I had my face in front of Beecher and while I was talking to him, he reached out and touched my hair and held it in his hand. He didn't pull it; he just seemed really interested in my hair. It was so sweet. Gary and Maggie said their goodbyes and left. I've said goodbye to Beecher so many times and each time someone else comes to see him and says goodbye knowing they may never see him again, I feel the pain and it hurts all over again. I walked Gary and Maggie out to their car and Gary hugged me for a long time and told me to hang in there. I told him that I am trying to be strong and that I appear to be so strong but I'm really not. I just have to be strong for everybody else. I keep wondering, when this is all going to end so I can get past this part of my life that is so filled with pain; but I know there is a lot of love there and some wonderful memories. I seem to cling to that to help me get through it. I was so emotional after Gary left, I cried the rest of the day.

When Gary got home, he told me this. "Just got home. I didn't say anything before I left because I was already crying. When Maggie went to the bathroom and you went to the kitchen, I was holding Beecher's right hand with my left hand and I leaned in and told him a couple of times that I loved him. He immediately took his other hand, the left one and grabbed my hand with it, holding my hand with both of his. He knew what I was saying to him. I knew you would want to know. He is still there somehow and does still understand some things. It surprised me when he did." I couldn't stop crying when Gary told me this.

~

September 21

I met the caseworker at TLC. Jerri said Beecher's oxygen level was 90 which is kind of low. It should be 91 and above. His blood pressure was 110/75 which is good. She addressed his bedsore issues and put new bandages on them. The sore behind his right knee looks pretty bad and also the one on his bottom. They don't seem to be getting better. I know they do the best that they can and Diane, the caregiver, always puts an ace bandage around his knees to help.

~

September 23

Today I took Beecher an ice cream cone from Dairy Queen. His eyes got really big when I showed it to him; however, he had a hard time eating it as he couldn't get his mouth open and he couldn't stick out his tongue to lick it.

I finally put the ice cream in a bowl and fed it to him. He didn't eat all of it and he seemed to be uncomfortable for some reason today. He felt very warm to me and I asked Diane if he had a fever and she said no. Maybe it was just the sun shining through the window.

But he did moan several times when she was changing the bandage on his leg. I didn't stay too long as I had some errands to run and had a guy from Nevada energy coming to give me an energy assessment at my home.

~

September 24

Had a great time at my high school reunion at The Orleans. Good to see my old friends. Afterwards, my friends and I went down to the lounge to watch Amy performing with her new band. It was a great evening and fun to get out for a change.

~

September 27

Beecher had his appointment with Dr. Léger today. BP was 100/67 which is the lowest I've ever seen it. No weight taken today (too hard to get him standing on the scale). Beecher was very attentive to Dr. Léger and his assistant Maileen. Dr. Léger took a 30 second video of Beecher that he wants to use for training purposes for physicians. He asked my permission to use Beecher's name when he is doing training or at different events. Of course, I agreed to it.

He also told me that he has followed Beecher more than any other patient he's ever had. Dr. Léger had only been at the Brain Center for one year when he started seeing Beecher three years ago. At that time, he diagnosed Beecher with PPA and FTD and he has followed him throughout this illness to the end. He said he had a special interest in Beecher because of that and also because of the artistic part of him that was able to produce the paintings he has done. He told me that he had heard that I was making a book for Beecher with his watercolors. He asked me if I had an editor for it. I then told him I had made the book myself through Shutterfly. I had Beecher hand him a copy of the book that I made specifically for Dr. Léger. He felt much honored. He told me that publishing a book was very expensive and there may be some funding that he could help me to get more books published. He said he couldn't promise anything but he would do what he could. I thought that was very nice of him. I also told him I've been writing a journal for three years and he asked me if I was going to write a book. I said I'm planning on it. He said he may be able to help me with that as well. So, we'll see.

He asked if he could do another pet scan on Beecher's brain since it's been three years and I said yes. I just did not want to bring him back again for another visit. Dr. Léger set it up to have it done that day. I will get a copy of it when it is finished on a disc. The doctor also wanted to wean Beecher off the Seroquel as he said it may help with some stiffness in his body.

After the visit I walked outside with Dr. Léger and I asked him what his prognosis was at this time. He said Beecher may go on like this for several more months. He said if he gets pneumonia to not give him antibiotics just let his body do what needs to be done. He also said to continue all other meds that Hospice had prescribed including morphine to be given to him every four hours as needed for pain. He told me he will be in touch with me about the books. This would be Beecher's last visit with Dr. Léger. His primary diagnosis now is Corticobasal Degeneration (CBS) with FTD and PPA as the secondary diagnosis. Physical changes include more difficulties with swallowing requiring thickener for fluids. He now needs assistance of four people instead of two at last visit. He has been wheelchair bound since July, more rigid now, can still follow simple commands but has a hard time executing actions. Pressure sores on back of knees and buttocks persists. He is now unable to play games on his iPad but he still enjoys listening to music via headset. Doctor said he is currently in end stage, totally mute and unable to ambulate. His FAST track (which is the level for criteria for hospice which he already qualified for) is now estimated at 7E due to his body stiffness. His overall prognosis is likely less than six months. After the visit; they took him down the hall to do a CT scan. Also Dr. Léger said that the RJ article and video should be coming out this week during the AFTD awareness week. There will be a Zumba event at the Brain Center on October 2nd which is Beecher's 62nd birthday. There will be a five-dollar donation with all the proceeds going to research. The CT scan report did indicate a chronic change (moderate volume loss in the frontal lobes and prominence of the anterior portions) and showed a somewhat frontal prominence of volume loss, which could be the sequence of Pick's disease. (Interpretation of the Cleveland Clinic Imaging Institute)

September 28

I met Melinda the caseworker at the group home today. Beecher's blood pressure was 140/85 which is higher than it's been in a while. She also measured his arm and said it was only 24 inches around. She said that is quite a loss as it was measured in July at 27 and then again at 26. So, he's lost another two inches since July due to eating less and still dropping weight. She measured the bed sore on his bottom. Last week when she measured it was 1.5 x 1.5. Today it was 3 ½ x 1 1/2 which is a two-inch increase since last Wednesday. Not good. Bedsores are very difficult to heal. The problem is that if the infection gets into his bones, it will most likely end his life. I got a message from MacKenzie regarding the interview. She said she heard a rumor that the article and video will be released sometime during the AFTD awareness week. She said Pash, the reporter, is really excited about the piece and so is she.

September 30

Visited Beech today. Fed him his lunch and clipped his fingernails. His fingernails grow so fast. I have a hard time clipping his nails as he cannot straighten out his fingers but I managed to get them clipped anyway. It just takes me longer. He got a birthday card from Nathan Adelson. Beecher opened it and looked at it and acted like he was reading it, but I just don't know any more whether he can read or not. He only ate half of his lunch today. One of the caregivers said a month ago he was eating a full bowl of food and now he only eats about half. However, he did eat all of his ice cream, as usual. I talked to the girls about his birthday party on Sunday at 2:30. They are going to have it outside on the patio and all the residents and caregivers will be there. That will be nice. I was there about two hours. He had his eyes open most of the time today. I know he is getting tired of all this. I pray for him every night that this will be over soon for all of us.

～

October 2

Beecher's 62nd Birthday! I dropped a German Chocolate Cake off at the Group Home. Diane told me he had cried in his sleep a lot the night before. Wish I knew what he was crying about, whether he has bad dreams, is in pain or just tired of this horrible disease. I cried all the way as I drove to the "Food for Thought" Awareness Week event at the Brain Center. It was a Zumba event to raise money for FTD. On the way I heard the song, "I Need You Now" by Lady Antebellum, which is the ringtone on my phone for Beecher. My heart just breaks for him when I hear that. I sat and talked to Lisa Radin. Dr. Léger was also there and spoke for a few minutes. One of the girls from my support group spoke for a while about her husband who has FTD. He is only 46. They have three children. When I think how bad I've had it, I don't know how I could have done it while raising three children.

After the event, I went back to the group home for Beecher's party. Amy, Michelle, Cole and Frisco came as well as good friends, Dave and Anita. The Director made some Long Noodles and Michelle brought some eggrolls. All the residents and care givers joined in the party. The Director, Francesca, even sang Happy Birthday to Beecher. He opened all the cards and seemed to like the toys, which are mostly what he got except for two t-shirts from Amy. It was a great day and he was very observant and seemed to know it was his birthday. Got some great pictures and videos. I was going to stay and snuggle with him, but they were going to keep him up for another hour, and I was exhausted. I will have to go visit him some day late in the day, since I promised I would lay with him for a while.

～

October 3

Dr. Léger messaged me and asked me if he could use Beecher's name and share his story at the Lunch and Learn this Wednesday at the Brain Center. I said, of course. He also asked me if I would say a few words and I agreed to that also.

~

October 5

I went to the Lunch and Learn meeting at the Brain Center today. The Lunch and Learn meetings are recorded and are visible at remote locations including Pahrump and even Elko, Nevada. Dr. Léger was speaking. The whole subject was about Beecher from the beginning of his illness up until today. He included information about observations and evaluations to determine how he was able to make this diagnosis about Beecher. He included several pictures of Beecher's watercolors and talked about how unusual it was that he had the ability to paint so well. He showed several of Beecher's painting during the presentation. He did a PowerPoint presentation and at the end he showed a 30 second video that he took of Beecher in his office last week. That video is available on YouTube and the link is at the end of my book. I got a little choked up when I saw it even though I was there when he took the video. I did not know that I was going to react that way. Some of the things he discussed were about Corticobasal Degeneration and Progressive Supranuclear Palsy which both have Parkinsonism's which Beecher now has, such as early falls and movement disorders and stiffness in joints. He was rigid on the right side called cog willing which is a Parkinson symptom.

The doctor talked about how unusual it was for Beecher to be interested in watercolor but that part of the brain did not appear to be affected by FTD. He also said that 10% of all dementia is in younger people with FTD and that 40% is genetic. In Beecher's case his shrinkage of the brain was evident in his anti-social behavior, stuttering, yes/no answers, no longer cooking and the fact that at one time he had been an inspirational speaker and had lost his speech, and developed obsessive behaviors and had gained over 30 lbs. since his first visit in May of 2013.

Dr. Léger went on to talk about how FTD is analyzed to determine if someone has it. They use what they call possible or probable indications; if someone has certain indications of symptoms that it is possible or probable, they have FTD. Usually, three out of six things determine the outcome. In Beecher's case, they judged by the hands on the clock and numbers not being in the right place, the fact he drove over spikes in a driveway and he knows better because he is in construction, and he used several F words when asked to say eleven words that start with the letter F and two of them are F words you don't usually say to a doctor, if you know what I mean. He scored six out of six things that determined it was not only possible but probable as well that he had FTD. The changes in Beecher occurred on a scale of months of doctor's visits that were noticed over a period of time.

Starting with 16 months after onset he had falls, choking, change in bowel habits, voice volume dropped to a whisper and his body was becoming rigid.

At 22 months, he was more isolated as he played with his iPad and the game Angry Birds all day. He had no spontaneous speech, had developed PSP and CBS, was motionless and unable to move unless asked, and his eye movements were restricted.

At 28 months, he was more passive, obsessive with urination, nearly mute, choking and drooling.

At 33 months, his only communication was thumbs-up or down. He was unable to use utensils to eat. He needed help dressing, and couldn't look up or down. His head and chest were rigid as if one body part instead of two, as if stuck for the rest of his days. It is customary for these Lunch and Learn lectures to be recorded and made available online for interested individuals to see. These links are posted at the end of this book under Resources.

After the presentation, Dr. Léger asked me to get up and speak. I didn't realize how emotional I was but I got up and said how I felt about the disease and how it had taken away every good thing about Beecher. I was emotional but I was able to get through a couple minutes of speaking. I thanked Dr. Léger and his staff for all the help that I received over the last three years. Afterwards, his nurse Nancy came up and hugged me and another lady who was hosting the meeting. Another lady and her husband came over to me and the lady hugged me and told me I was a very strong woman. That made me feel good as I looked at her husband and he looked like he might have had some form of dementia.

On my way home, I stopped to see Beecher. He was in bed having his nap. I crawled up on his bed and lay with him for about fifteen minutes. I think he liked it. As he kept grabbing my hand, I talked to him and told him how much I loved him and that I wish I could change everything that has happened to him. I cried and he had his eyes open most of the time so I know he was listening to me. I also told him that someday soon he would get to go to the other side where he's always talked about going, and then he will be out of all the pain that he is in now. It was such an emotional day that by the time I got home I felt drained.

I talked to the caseworker Jerrie after I got home. She was there for her visit with Beecher today. She said his vitals were all good. His bed sores are having a hard time healing. She ordered some blue booties that have straps on them so they can keep those on his feet and ankles because of the bedsores instead of the ace bandages. The Hospice doctor also took him off of Hydroxyzine and started him on another drug called Lorazepam .5 mg. It will help with his anxiety and also his breathing as Diane said sometimes, he seems to have trouble breathing.

October 6

I got a message from Dr. Léger thanking me for coming and speaking at the Lunch and Learn. He said he thinks the attendees were, as he was, very moved by my comments. He said they are very fortunate that I felt comfortable letting him tell Beecher's story, because it is compelling and really helps others to understand the disease. He also said that it is customary for these lectures to be recorded and made available online for interested individuals to see and they would be also be available on YouTube.

October 8

Our friend Bret came to visit Beecher and me. He came to the house and picked me up. I gave him a copy of the watercolor book I made for Beecher and also a mug. He was so overwhelmed at the thought. He said he wanted to sit and look at it later. When we arrived at the group home, Beecher seemed to be glad to see Bret. Bret told me that Beecher and he had a very spiritual relationship. (I did not know that!) I tried feeding Beecher his lunch but after about six bites he seemed to be in pain and was having trouble swallowing. He took a few sips of water, but that didn't seem to help. He squinted his eyes and moaned and it scared me. After several minutes of this, I asked Diane, the caregiver to come help me. After several more minutes, he finally seemed okay. I didn't give him any more food. Bret asked me if he could have a few minutes alone with Beecher, so naturally I said "sure."

I walked into the kitchen for a few minutes and then finally sat in a chair by the table where the other residents eat. I had an amazing experience while I was sitting there. One of the sweet ladies, named Miriam, who is 93 years young and a resident there, (who is also hard of hearing and I always talk to when I go to visit), came over to me. She is very agile for her age and except for her memory and her hearing, she seems absolutely fine. She saw that I was in stress about Beecher because of his incident with the food. She put her arm around me and hugged me, kissed me on the cheek and told me it was going to be okay. She did this several times and I thanked her for comforting me. When I looked into her eyes, I said "If my mother were still alive, she would be the same age as you." She would have been 92. I told her I saw my mother's eyes in her eyes and the glorious look on her face as she smiled and said once again, "It's going to be okay." She also kept stroking my hair. This was such a comforting moment in my life to know that my mom was watching over us. (Even though Beecher never got to meet her as she died several years before I met him.) Miriam said Beecher was such a sweet man and it was sad that he was going through this at such a young age. She always waved to him from across the room and he would wave back. Sometimes, she would come over to him and run her hand over his head to comfort him as well. She did this on many occasions when I was there. (Little did I know until this day, that she was the angel that was sent to watch over him, when I wasn't there.) I asked her how many years she had been married and she said 37 years. When I asked her how old her husband was when he died (just assuming he died), she said, "You know, I don't remember. I don't think I have a very good memory anymore, at least that is what my doctor told me and that's why I live here now." She smiled and laughed so nonchalantly. All the residents, including the caregivers really love Beech and they watch over him. I am so blessed as he is getting the best care possible. Bret finally waved at me to come back and sit with him and Beecher. He thanked me for allowing him to spend that time with him. He is such a sweet lovable guy. We spent about four hours visiting him.

When we got back to my house, Bret starting telling me about his visit alone with Beech. He said he hoped I didn't mind, that he had a very "go to the light now" talk with him. He told him that I would be okay. I started crying and Bret put his arms around me, hugged me and let me get my tears out. I thanked him for talking to Beech and sharing the talk with me. I had been having a hard time having that conversation with him. I know it's time to let go and believe me, I have been trying, but it is the hardest thing to do. As each day slips by, I see him declining and see the pain in his eyes. I know he wants to leave this planet earth, but it is in God's plan, not mine. I also told Bret that I didn't think Beech would even make it to his 62nd birthday but he is strong willed (probably just wanted a few more toys before he left, LOL.) I told Bret that I was so afraid that Beech would die on my birthday which is next Saturday, October 15 when I turn 70 years old. I have always had this feeling because for many years of my life the time on the clock mostly said 10:15 when I looked at it. I always felt that was supposed to signify something, besides my birthday. I was afraid that I would always feel sad on that day and could never really celebrate my birthday, but instead feel sorrow that he died on that day. Bret said the most profound thing to me. He said," Nancy, don't think that way. Think of it as a gift you gave to him on your birthday to let him go." I started crying again and thanked him for such a wonderful way to look at it. Words of wisdom, that I could not see. What a remarkable remembrance to have of my beloved, that he would choose to depart this world on my birthday, so I would never forget him; to free the pain that has been trapped inside his mind and body for so long. As I write this, I pray that the time will come soon and he can have that "out of body experience" that he has wanted for so long.

As Bret left, he promised to stay in touch and said he would always be here for me and Beech. I believe he will. He gave me a most generous birthday gift and told me to promise to spend it on myself and no one else. But the most precious gift were his words of wisdom and his compassion that will help me survive the end of this journey as I prepare myself for Beecher's death.

Bret and I have texted many times after he left today. He told me that his visit meant the world to him, and that his heart was full of love for both of us. He said that I was the best thing to ever happen to Beech and that Beech is so blessed to have me. He said he didn't quite know how to put into words the gratitude in his heart for my trust and allowing him to talk to Beech heart to heart. He thanked me again for the book and said he will treasure it forever. I responded by telling him that his friendship means a great deal to me and I hope we remain friends for life. I sent him the link to the YouTube presentation that Dr. Léger did on Wednesday at the Brain Center about Beech. He said he would be sure to watch it. He said his wife looked at the book and she absolutely loved it. He advised me to make sure that my girls go visit Beech this week as he feels his time is coming near. He told me what an amazing person I was. I told him, you do what you have to do for the ones you love. Somehow you gain the strength and courage to travel this rocky road. I do believe it comes from God and I'm thankful for all my family and amazing friends that I have in my life. Bret said the next time I see Beech to give him a kiss from him. He was sure he would get a chuckle out of the kiss. LOL!

~

October 9

I woke up this morning feeling so loved and so blessed. "I Got This, God!" I said to myself. I can do this! Amy went to visit Beech and she facetimed me. He kept putting his hand out toward me, like he was trying to touch me. It was so endearing. Amy took him some coconut water and some eggnog and she said he drank the eggnog down without stopping! He never ceases to amaze me! I always try to think of things to take him that I know he loves, like pudding, yogurt, watermelon juice, and milk shakes. I had forgotten about eggnog as he always looked forward to this season when it's available as he really loved it. My brother Ricky and his wife Christine took me to dinner for my birthday since they will be out of town on my birthday. Had a nice dinner and visit with them.

~

October 10, Columbus Day

Went to visit Beech. He was very still and had his eyes closed for most of the visit. However, I told him I had a great big kiss for him from Bret. As I neared him to kiss him, his lips puckered. I planted a big one on him. I then told him I had a kiss for him too, and he did the same thing. It was the first time in a long time that I actually felt him kissing me back. It was so special. I texted Bret later that I had given Beech the kiss from him and how he had responded with both of our kisses. I told him we were in competition. Bret texted back that he had a feeling that I was going to win! LOL! I sat with Beech for a while and at one point as I was holding his hand, I told him I was there and would always be there for him. As he had his eyes closed most of the time, I wasn't sure if he was sleeping or just resting. I told him, "If he knew I was there, to give me a thumbs-up," and immediately he did. It was a quick response and I was so glad I asked him. He is still in there and my heart swelled with love for him. I left to go to lunch with my sister, Patti. He had been having a slight fever that was not always going down with Tylenol, so the hospice was called. It was weird as his head and chest and underarms were really hot, but his cheeks, arms and legs were very cold. I was going to go back later but called instead and the caregivers said the hospice doctor had ordered a new medication to help his fever and his pain. I think they are giving him morphine every four hours too.

October 11

Jerri, the new case manager, called me and said she had visited Beecher to give him a suppository since he hadn't had a bowel movement in several days. She also said that Diane has been taking his temperature on a more regular basis and said his temp last night was 107! Jerri said that was probably not accurate and I agreed. Since Diane is hard to understand sometimes, maybe she meant 100.7. Anyway, his temp is going down and I am going to meet her there tomorrow to visit him. I will get a better understanding of what's going on. I talked to MacKenzie in regards to the article and video that was to be published several weeks ago. Apparently, it had been pushed back. She said that sometimes happens with larger articles like Beecher's and she would let me know when she has a better idea of when the article will run.

October 12

Went to visit Beecher and to meet Jerri, the case manager from hospice. I was feeding Beech before she got there and he was having a hard time swallowing. He was trying to cough up some of the food and he seemed like he was in pain again like the other day. He also had another bedsore; this one on his ear. She checked his heart and lungs and said that she didn't hear any congestion so that was good. The girls took him into the room so she could check his bedsores on his bottom. They were still about the same and he had a new spot. Also, the one behind his knee is starting to scab over. So that was good. Blood pressure was 134/67. After she finished her assessment, she said that if his pain got any worse, they could put him on more morphine. She called the doctor and asked if the fever was infection could they could give Beech antibiotics. I told her no I did not want him to have antibiotics and also his doctor said no as well. He would not want to live like that. She said she would put an alert in his chart that no life saving measures should be considered.

After she left, I sat with him and held his hand and told him that if he was ready to go, I would be OK. I do not want him to be like this and I didn't want him to suffer anymore. I told him I knew Bret had talked to him about this. I had taken his laser light and plugged it in his room. I turned it on even though it was daytime and he could see the green spots on the ceiling and his eyes got very big several times. I also pushed the button on his new dog toy I had gotten and set it to play fifteen minutes of lullaby music. He seemed very content. Before I left, I talked to him again and asked if he wanted me to kiss him. He had his eyes open and as I started to kiss his lips, he moved to accept my kiss. I asked him if I could kiss him one more time again and I told him how much I loved him. It was a very sad day for me but I knew the words needed to be said and I didn't want him to struggle and be in pain anymore. I told that to the nurse as well that I'm ready to let him go. She understood and said that she would always check with me first. P.S. She said she thinks he is transitioning. He is pretty much confined to his bed now in his room.

~

October 13

I went to watercolor class and finished my Christmas card which was a picture of One Lonely Lovebird on a Limb in honor of Beech and then went to visit him for a short time.

~

October 14

Went to lunch with the girls from LVHS and afterwards I went to visit Beech. He's not eating or drinking.

October 15, Today is my birthday

Went to visit Beech. Diane, the caregiver was giving him a Starbucks Cappuccino and he really seemed to be enjoying it and drank it all. My daughters took me out to dinner for my big 70th birthday at the Tuscany Grill. As always, we had a wonderful time. Amy gave me a picture of Beecher and me on canvas. Made me cry as always.

October 16

My grandson Tyler and Michelle came by to visit Beech. I met them there. It was a short visit and not much to say but that Beecher is definitely declining more and more each day.

October 17

I woke up at 3:20 a.m. and couldn't get back to sleep. At 3:40 a.m. Diane from TLC called me and said Beecher woke up with a sore throat and said she had called the Hospice because Beecher was having a hard time swallowing. She was crying and said I should come over right away. So of course, I got dressed and drove right over. I called Amy and she met me there. She only lives three minutes away from the home.

When I got there the nurse was there and she checked his vitals and said they were good and his breathing was ok. He had a slight fever. She increased his morphine. She assured me they would continue to give him morphine to keep him comfortable until end of life even if he was comatose. He's is not very attentive today and eating very little and not drinking much water. I stayed with him for a while and then went back home to bed. I had a flying dream about Beecher and me. He was flying but he started falling down. We were holding hands and I told him it was okay and that he could try again. I woke up at 8:10 with the phone ringing.

October 18

We had a gig at TLC to celebrate me and Beecher's birthdays. Yes, performers included the one and only Amy Sung and Stephanie Calvert, plus Bucky Heard from the Righteous Brothers, Rick Duarte, John Wedermeyer and Shaun De Graff. Of course, Michelle, Cole, Tyler, my granddaughter Leah, Fran, Anabelle, Dave & Anita came too. It was a real treat for the other patients and the caregivers as well. Amazing day! Beech was very attentive and really seemed to enjoy the music and the people although he seemed a little uncomfortable. It was a huge success and we were able to pull it off on time like we wanted to.

October 19

Got a call from the Hospice caregiver, Jerrie, to meet her at the Home at 8 am to discuss Beecher's progression. I went back at 11 am with my friend Belinda. My oldest granddaughter Leah stopped by to visit also. We stayed awhile and then Belinda and I went to catch a quick lunch to celebrate my birthday.

October 20

Hospice called around 9 am and said I should come soon so I left immediately. She said Beecher is transitioning and it won't be long. He is close to the end. I called my daughters to come to the home. They arrived shortly. Our friend, Janon was supposed to come sit with him that night while my girls and I went to an "Elks Old Timer's Dinner" at the Elks Lodge that night to present Beecher with a 30-year pin. I knew we would not make it and Janon offered to come by and say her last goodbye to him and to be there for us. Janon came in the evening. She sat and talked to him while we were in the room. She is a very spiritual woman as well as a psychic. They have a very special deep spiritual connection. After a while she said Beecher is having a hard time as he wants to go, but he also wants to stay. She finally said he wanted to be alone with us girls only. My granddaughters, Suzie and Bekkah were in town and they stopped by shortly to see him and say goodbye to him.

It was a long day and a long night but I did not leave his side except to use the bathroom. Beecher and I had always felt that no one should die alone and I was determined to be at his side as he took his last breath. As the room was very small and the hospital bed was not very big, we had the caregivers bring in a bench and my girls and I took turns lying next to him on the bed and the other two lying on the bench. We cuddled and held Beecher and talked to him about how beautiful heaven was going to be and how he would no longer be in pain. He would be at peace and that our little Cammie who had passed away in 2013 would be waiting for him and also his two brothers and his mother and his dad. Most of the time he had his eyes open and looked back and forth to the left and right often looking into my eyes. We got very little sleep as we all dozed off and on. I kept my hand on his chest near his heart so I could feel if his breathing was changing. We surrounded him with love and peace and played some of his special music. Lying next to him and cuddling him, I know he knew I was there with us girls and he felt the love.

October 21

We got very little sleep if any at all. Sometime around 4 or 5 am, I noticed Beecher's breathing had changed and I could hear soft breathing. The girls opened their eyes when I told them and we prepared ourselves for the end. Diane came in at some point to give him some morphine. I waved her away because I knew it was almost over and she knew it too. His skin had started turning purple (called mottling) which is a sign that death is near. The Hospice nurse had explained to me that the heart wants to be the last thing to stop and so all the other organs in the body start shutting down to save the heart.

The phone calls from his stepdaughter, Kim, granddaughter's, Suzie and Bekkah, and my friend Mie, wore on as the morning slowly crept past. Michelle's best friend Andrea came over and brought us some breakfast from McDonalds' as we hadn't eaten anything since the day before. She stayed in the room with us and got to witness his passing. Amy had posted on Facebook and a lot of people were already sending their condolences. Lots of sad feelings and more music. The end was coming very quick. Around 11:30 am my grandson Justin called to say goodbye. He was the last of the grandkids to say goodbye. Beecher must have been waiting for that call. Immediately after, his breathing changed again. The rise and fall of his chest as the lungs diminished more. The end was imminent. I felt the angels around me. When I was fourteen, I had an angel experience where an angel had appeared to me and I had always felt her presence throughout my life. Also, thirteen years ago when my brother-in-law passed, I was in the room with him and his ex-daughter-in-law. I had awakened that morning knowing I needed to go visit him that day. As my brother-in-law lay there dying, I got into a conversation with the daughter-in–law about angels and she said she wasn't sure they were real. I started telling her my experience, and at that moment, I felt that angel coming into the room from an open window and I said ,"I know they are real" and at that second my brother-in-law took his last breath. That feeling that I had that morning was that I was supposed to help him pass over. I truly believe he heard me and he felt the angels coming to take him away and he needed to hear a confirmation.

I did not see the angels today with Beech but I felt their presence as they guided me as I shared my last words to him. At one point, Amy was sitting closest to him and I ask her to change seats with me. We played "Time" by Sir Lawrence Oliver. I spoke to Beecher gently as the words flowed directly from my heart. I told him how much we all loved him. How brave he had been. That he was my hero and that I had never loved anyone like I loved him. I asked his forgiveness for anything that I had ever said bad or done to him. I apologized to him for my feelings sometimes when I couldn't handle the situation of his disease. That it wasn't him. That I wasn't mad at him, but I was mad at the disease. He continued to stare through to me throughout this period of time and I could see in his eyes that he knew what I was saying. I told him it was OK to go; that Cammie and my mom and his mom and his brothers were all waiting for him. I told him I would be OK and Amy and Michelle would be OK and they would watch over me as he had taught them to do. I told him he was going to a better place, a more beautiful place where he would be without pain and suffering. I told him he was such a strong warrior and that he had lived a good life and helped so many people. I told him I had so many wonderful memories of him and he taught me so much and that he had taught me courage and strength and he had given so much to me and to others. That he had been a father to my girls when he didn't have to but because he wanted to and I respected him for that and always will.

I remember at one point, Michelle said," I never thought this would be so beautiful." The passing of one's life from this world into the next. That's when my world came to an end and I felt his chest, his heartbeat slowing down and as his eyes looked at me one last time, I felt him and heard him as he took his last breath. Not wanting him to go but knowing I finally had to let him go as I had told him I was ready to do. I wished him well on his journey and told him I would never forget him, that he was the love of my life and that I would always remember him. As he took his last breath at 12:05 pm, I felt the life go out of him. I thanked God for taking him so gently and for allowing me and my daughters to be there as he crossed over into the hands of God and where Cammie, our dog and all the others that were waiting to celebrate his arrival back home. My heart aches for him as I write these words but I am so blessed to have been there and mostly because my daughters were there as well. I knew he did not want to die alone and I said that I would be there to the end and I was as I had promised. As sad as it was, it was an experience that I will always hold dear to my heart. And the fact that the girls were there to experience it with me. To watch one's life end in such a beautiful way, I could only describe his death as beautiful. Somewhere during this time, we had played the song "Jealous of the Angels." I know Beecher would be watching over us. Throughout the last 26 hours or so, he had his eyes open most of the time looking at us and very seldom closing his eyes as if he wanted to see us so he could remember us the way we were. Even Jerrie had told me on Thursday that he had his eyes closed before I arrived yesterday and as soon as he knew I was in his room his eyes fluttered open and he never closed them after. He was waiting for me to be there to hold his hand and to help him crossover. His wings were ready but my heart was not.

The next few hours were somewhat of a blur. Justin and Bethany arriving, the grandkids coming back to say their last goodbye. Phone calls, the coroner arriving, Kennedy (Amy's ex-husband) and Stephanie going to get us food to eat. Did not want to see the coroner take his body away. Packing his clothes and all of his belongings to take back to our home. The Cinderella tie-dyed T-shirt that Amy had given him which was the last thing he wore before he died. I asked the coroner to please take it off and bring it to me before they took his body away. The dampness of the sweat on the t-shirt as he passed from this world to the next brought me comfort. The goodbyes to the caregivers especially Diane who had taken her role as caregiver so emotionally and comfortingly and the love that she felt for him for someone she had only met eight months prior. Remembering that she came in the night before to give him a shot of morphine and she was so emotional it took her several minutes to put the medication into his mouth. Miriam who is now like another mother. The times that she came into the room to give us love and comfort and kissing me, Michelle and Amy. The pictures that she brought into the room to show us of her husband who had died many years before. She shared them with us. I felt the sadness from all the caregivers and all the residents that made my visits to him so loving and so kind. I know they will all miss him too. Leaving the home for the last time with Beecher being there but promising that I would return to visit. I will be sure to do that because they were his friends and caregivers until the end. God, please help me to remember that promise as they were also instrumental in the passing months when I was not there to comfort and care for Beech.

Called the mortuary to alert them that Beecher has passed. They will notify the local pathologist to go to the mortuary as soon as possible to remove his brain and get it sent to Cleveland Clinic within 24 hours.

His brain donation. Hopefully he will help others and find a cure so that no one and no families will have to bear the results of this horrible disease that has taken him away from us.

The drive home was a blur…

A call from my son Steve to give me his condolences.

Arriving at home knowing that my life was about to change.

A life without Beech.

Remembering the words, I used to say. "Life's a Beech and then you marry one."

Beecher was always such a kid at heart and I used to say he may grow older but he will never grow up. And then saying I raised all my other kids and now I will spend the rest of my life raising Beecher. I guess I put that up to the universe never realizing that I would be doing exactly that someday. And that is exactly what I did for the last four years as our life changed with this dreadful disease that attacked his body. The disease that came in the night like a thief to take away all the good things about him. His speech, his personality and the loving caring person whose mission in life was to save everybody else. But the only person he could not save was himself.

EPILOGUE—2016-2017
LIFE AFTER BEECH

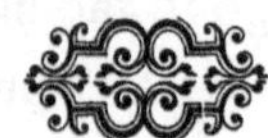

As I walked into our home knowing that I would never see Beecher's face again until some point in my life when I will join him in heaven and be with him for eternity. Feeling so glad that I wasn't walking into an empty house as he has been gone from this home, our home for over a year. Really glad that I had gone through his clothing and his other personal belongings, his tools, and his books. Everything that I had taken the time to do to make this transition easier for me in the end. Knowing and feeling that his life had a purpose and he had served that purpose here on earth and now he's with God and he is up there to help save so many souls. God must've loved him enough to allow him to live here on earth. As he was born a baby, he arrived home as a baby. Through the transition of this disease, it may be that it was meant to be that way. Only God knows.

The heartfelt cries that I was able to feel when I first was alone at home as I sobbed my heart out.

My girls coming to be with me and spending the first night with me loving and comforting me and sharing the experience of his last day on earth.

Phoebe, Amy's cat and my grand kitty is here with us and being such a good girl.

The sensor lights that came on in the night in the bathroom while I slept as Amy witnessed them coming on eight times. Michelle moving to the guestroom because I was keeping her awake with my snoring.

Michelle coming back into my bedroom and sitting on the other side of the bed as we talked and reminisced some more as Amy told her about the night lights coming on in the bathroom. After a while, Amy fell back asleep. As Michelle and I talked, Michelle said she saw and I also saw out of the corner of my eye, one of the sensor lights going off in the bathroom. Michelle had never even seen it come on but we both witnessed it going off. The sensor lights only come on when there is movement in the bathroom. We both felt it was Beecher's presence.

~

October 22

I got a call from Cleveland Clinic in Ohio around 8 am. They had already received Beecher's brain.

Going through his belongings that we brought home from the TLC Home and deciding which things we wanted to keep and which ones we wanted to give to the people who loved him. The toys that will go to the grandkids and the great grandkids, the coloring books, the paints. All the things that he held dear to him that were a part of his last few days and years of his life.

The talk with my sister Linda later in the morning. She talked about the last seven minutes of heaven and how she had heard about the energy that remained when someone left this earth. The fact that the lights coming on and off during the night were letting us know it was our sign that he was OK and that he had arrived safely in heaven.

All the heartfelt messages I read from people that loved and respected Beecher so much. The people that I didn't even know he had helped. Over 900 messages in the last two or three days since this journey started coming to an end.

~

October 23

Waking up this Sunday morning. Taking the last t-shirt Beecher wore and putting it on me. The tie-dyed one that Amy had given him some time ago. The sweat and the tears during his last few days. The tears that I dried from his eyes on those last two days of his passing. Yesterday I saw two love birds on a limb. Today there is only one.

~

October 26

Called Dr. Léger. He did not know Beecher had passed. He never received my message. Nice talk with him. I invited him to the Celebration of Life on Sunday. I also invited Nancy his nurse who was able to attend but Dr. Léger could not because of his schedule.

~

October 27

My sister Linda arrived from California to console me and help with the Celebration of Life.

~

October 28

I got an email from MacKenzie sending her condolences. She also spoke with Dr. Léger yesterday and let me know she had also reached out to Pash for an update on when the article will run. Pash sent her condolences as well and apologized for the delay. She hopes to run it sometime next week. *Note: (It actually got pushed to April 2017 to coincide with the Power of Love Gala, which got much more attention.) More on that later.*

I went to the movies with my sisters, Linda and Patti. I don't even remember what movie we saw.

October 30

Beecher's Celebration of Life was held at the Elks Lodge. My brother Donny and his wife Madie came from California to attend as well as my brother Ricky and his wife Chris and my sister Patti who live here in Las Vegas. What better place to have it as he was a member for 30 years and we were the first couple to ever get married at this Lodge. Included was beautiful live music by Amy, Rick Duarte, Shaun DeGraff, John Encino and a special performance by Stephanie Calvert singing "Jealous of the Angels." John talked about Beecher's dedication to the Lodge and honored him in a moment of silence for the 11th hour. The Lodge presented his 30-year pin and donated the charity box money to me. In the beautiful brochure I made, I included Beecher's Favorite Beecherism's which included "It is what it is," and Words Beecher lived by which included "Life on Life's Terms," and my favorite saying " Life's a Beech and Then You Marry One." Also included was the "Serenity Prayer" from his NA program. In 2003 Beecher wrote his own eulogy. I had found it with some of his poems and of course, I included that. Beecher was a poet and had written many poems in his life. I had saved all of them and plan to make a book of his poems sometime in the near future. The Eulogy goes like this:

It is not death itself that diminishes:
But the passing of this reality into memory

To the loss of touch, word, smell and interactions.
These things we miss
These things we took for granted.
In this memory, let us not forget
What we have

So, we never again forget
Even the most insignificant moments
For the rest of our lives.

How appropriate was this eulogy? It was as if he knew years before that he was going to suffer from FTD. The wording of "loss of touch, word, smell, and interactions" and "the passing of this reality into memory."

Another poem he wrote in 1998 I included goes like this:

Ensign Half Mast by Beecher Trail
5/11/98

The process of life is distinguished,
Separating the body and soul,
The part we play is remembering
Bring the two into whole.

Cause tomorrow's tomorrow
And yesterday was the past,
It's the insanity of thinking,
When we don't live today like the last.

Waiting for divine intervention,
Or these feelings to pass,
Are watercolors on a painting,
Life's dripping ensign half-mast.

This poem is in reference to a ship's flag being flown at half-mast when someone on the ship dies. Beecher had been in the Navy Seabees for five years. The fact that he used the words "watercolors on a painting" years before he started painting, amazes me. I often wonder if he knew something, before we did.

Amy made a beautiful video about his life. Over 200 people attended.

It was a wonderful tribute to the love of my life and I will never forget him.

Sometime after Beecher passed, Amy shared these notes she had written regarding his last 26 hours from the time we arrived at the home until his last breath.

Beecher's Ascension

After 26 hours of being by his side....

Janon's words through Beecher:

She said Beecher wanted us three to be there when he transitioned.

She asked if Beecher could be waiting for someone to call or visit him?

- He had a Warriors heart
- Tyler the Titan–referring to my youngest Grandson-Beecher's Godson
- Strings and moms dream
- He didn't want to be touched and moved
- Said he wasn't in any pain
- The sword and stone?
- He said it was time for her (Janon) to leave so we could be there with him.
- He saw mom (Nancy) as flowing blonde silver hair with lightening

After Justin called and spoke to him, only moments after, his breathing changed to a full chest breathing.

We all knew it was close. I noticed his forehead had the purplish mottling.

Mom spoke from her heart and the words poured out of her so beautifully and eloquently...

She apologized for ever making him feel like she was mad at him.

She told him she was smiling and that we would all be ok

We all encouraged him to let go and that we would all take care of each other, so don't hang on for us

We said, "Sail away, daddy."

We could feel each breath

It felt like labor (of giving birth), but the opposite.

We all held him and soon the breaths became more labored like a fish out of water and he was almost gasping but peacefully.

He stared into Moms eyes with so much love and trust, listening to every word as she poured out her heart and guided him. Me and Michelle expressed our love and appreciation for him for raising us as his own.

I thanked him for influencing both of my careers in massage and in music, and that I wouldn't have had the courage to especially go for my music career if it weren't for him. Michelle thanked him for always being there and helping her to grow into a woman and helping her through really tough times.

We felt every breath and as it slowed;

We kept saying "it's ok, you can go" "be free and go to the light" "don't be scared daddy" "fly like a bird."

You will always be in our hearts, your energy will never die...

You will get a new body and be whole again

You will be out of pain.

In such a strange way we were encouraging him and rooting him on to go.

It was what we all knew was best for him.

He stopped breathing momentarily at 12:03pm and even closed his eyes.

Then another time a minute later.

Then finally his last breath at 12:05 and his eyes reopened, his heart had stopped; it actually happened, his soul left his body. We cried over him.

It was a magical experience and he hung on for so long and his body was so frail and he no longer was who he wanted to be. I doubt he wanted to even live as long as he did but he hung in there for us and just the nature of his being, a survivor.

It was the most powerful and beautiful thing I have ever witnessed, the whole scene of love and transition.

He passed to the song "Wild Child" by Enya.

Benjamin Button - I thought of this movie about a baby that was born looking like an old man, and as he ages, he grows younger looking, like a clock ticking backwards.

Amy Lynn Sung

A Fallen Limb
Beecher A. Trail
October 2, 1954 – October 21, 2016

Author Unknown

A limb has fallen from the family tree
I keep hearing a voice that says…Grieve not for me.
Remember the best times, the laughter, the song,
The good life I lived while I was strong.
Continue my heritage; I'm counting on you,
Keep smiling and surely the sun will shine through.
My mind is at ease, my soul is at rest.
Remembering all, how I truly was blessed.
Continue traditions, no matter how small,
Go on with your life, don't' worry about falls.
I miss you all dearly, so keep up your chin,
Until the day comes, we're together again.

Also, this message I found seems appropriate to include as I'm sure he felt this way:

AFTERGLOW
(Credit and thanks to Helen Lowrie Marshall-author)

I'd like the memory of me to be a happy one.
I'd like to leave an afterglow of smiles when my life is done.
I'd like to leave an echo whispering softly down the ways.
Of happy times and laughing times and bright sunny days.
I'd like the tears of those who grieve, to dry before the sun.
Of happy memories that I leave when life is done.

If I could say one more thing to Beecher, it would be:

"It was not my choice to survive without you.
So, I chose to live and honor you."

I hope this book honors Beecher in the best way as he was a warrior and hero to all who had the good fortune of knowing him. My good friend Sandy's son, Scott stated on Facebook, "A family friend has gone home, Beecher Trail. What a funny, yet cool name, I thought when I first met the man. I haven't met another "Beecher" in my life since and if I had, I doubt he would have held up next to this one." Scott had worked for Beecher and he said the most important thing he learned from him was the value of being responsible and diligent on the job. He often thinks of that when he's being challenged with a job or tasks that suck.

A few additional things I'd like to share about Beecher, the person, (not the other one who was sick, I think you've heard enough about that person). The real Beecher Trail who touched so many lives. He taught me so much about love, courage and determination. He was intelligent, courageous, spiritual, a fighter, a warrior, a lover of animals, a martial artist, a watercolor artist, a wonderful father, loving husband, and a dedicated member of the Elks Lodge. He was also a man of many words. He often entertained us with his many imitations of the great John Wayne, W.C. Fields, Alf, and Elmer Fudd which he did very well. His favorite rendition was of Elmer Fudd doing Bugs Bunny singing Bruce Springfield's "Fire," Riding in my car, turn on the stereo, etc. When FTD struck him, he was in the prime of his life. Like a thief in the night, it stole everything good from the person he was; his speech, his personality and his social demeanor. He was sometimes a macho man and yet a child in so many ways and yet a powerful man with a huge heart and my soul mate.

My daughter Amy, whom he raised from the age of 11, says that he was such a fun loving, generous and hard-working man with a big personality. He was often strict with her, but she didn't appreciate it until she got older! LOL!

Amy and Michelle nicknamed him Beecher the Preacher because of the many wise quotes, funny expressions, and impressions, and the desire to help others that needed counseling even if they didn't think so! They always appreciated his nuggets of wisdom and his way with words. Sometimes he even had to literally sit on someone to make them listen and he liked to pick on Amy, sometimes by tickling her and Michelle to death! He was a fun dad and everyone loved him. Beecher, the Preacher, and sometimes referred to as Beecher, the Teacher. "If you always do what you've always done, you'll always get what you always got." With him it was always about making changes in yourself if you didn't like the way your life was going. Insanity is doing the same thing over and over and expecting different results. And of course, Keep on Keeping on. He was a kid at heart and he always made us laugh a lot.

My daughter Michelle said she was honored to have him in her life and she knows he is watching over us all, but she wishes he was still here to hug and hear his words of wisdom. She said she would love to have one more talk with him, one more hug, one more tickle or even one more lecture from him. Even though Michelle was 21 when I met him, he had a very strong influence on her life and her sons. She also said she was one of the lucky daughters and how she missed the long talks and lectures. He had a very deep voice and he always got the messages across and people sat up and really listened to him.

Many people that sent condolences after his passing, remarked on what a uniquely special person he was and said he had a profound influence on their lives. That he was full of wisdom and compassion and never wanted anything in return. He wanted nothing more than to see you succeed and do the right things. One man from his NA group remarked that Beecher helped him find a better way of life and the lessons Beecher taught him would remain with him for life.

My grandson Justin took Beecher to get a tattoo put on his arm in 2015 that said "I am not defined" with a red rose. He believed that you should give up defining yourself to yourself or others and to not be concerned with how others define you. When others define you, they are limiting themselves, so it's their problem. This was part of a statement from Eckhart Tolle who is an author of many books and a spiritual teacher whom Beecher respected very much. One of my granddaughters Suzie, remarked about his tattoo and said it couldn't be more perfect. He could no longer speak, but it does not define him. He can no longer take care of himself, but it does not define him. He is not defined by his illness, but by the great things he has done in his life. She said he always told her to stay in the now and how to be in the present and set all worries aside. Suzie was getting an ultrasound done when Beecher passed away. They were looking at the beautiful life inside of her when it happened. She felt very special and it helped her stay positive as there was some concern for her and her baby. (She gave birth to my third great grandson eight days later and named him Micah Legrand **Beecher** Meecham.) Note the middle name!

~

November 16

Went on a trip to the Grand Canyon and Sedona with my grandson Justin, his wife Bethany, Amy and Michelle. It was a very uplifting trip and very beautiful! Beecher and I had always wanted to go to the Grand Canyon but never got around to it. We had been to Sedona several times and it was one of our favorite places. We all took turns spreading his ashes in both places.

~

November 18

Daddy Beecher's journey – a message from Michelle

11/18-Reading Mommy's inscription to daddy Beecher's watercolor album-approximately 6:45 pm, I'm sitting in my chair in the living room under the ceiling fan light that I feel he has visited us a few times, I am about to read the inscription mommy wrote to me with her own hand-writing. I was holding daddy Beecher's angel wing urn necklace in my fingers, between my thumb, index and middle finger, (go figure the middle finger is included.)

As I'm reading the inscription and crying, I begin to feel this sensation coming from the urn, between my fingers, an energy I cannot really describe. Maybe a vibration, maybe a shift in the remains that I thought were solidly packed? This happened three times during reading mommy's inscription.

After a minute or two of finishing the reading of the inscription, and now, well into being a half an hour later, I shake the urn up and down, side to side in every direction and I do not experience any settlement of his remains, nor any vibration or shift of his remains. All that remains is the memory of the energy I was connected to when daddy Beecher was with me during my reading of mommy's inscription.

To my daughters, Michelle and Amy,

Sometimes life can be very painful,
It gets complicated at the worst of times and
Sometimes you have no idea

Where to go or what to do.
But that's why you have to keep going.
You have to push through all the hurts.
Work past all the painful memories.
Because sometimes the things that hurt the most
Are the things that make you stronger.
Don't ever let the light inside you dim.
Please stay strong.
Never stop yourself from living,
From loving, from hoping and dreaming.
You deserve it.

~

November 21

He's been gone a month today already. Reality still hasn't set in. I feel numb and still in shock.

Thought for the day and a reality check:

Heart and Soul

"The death of a spouse or partner is different than other losses, in the sense that it literally changes every single thing in your world going forward. When your spouse dies, the way you eat changes. The way you watch TV changes. Your friend circle changes (or disappears entirely.) Your family dynamic/life changes (or disappears entirely.) Your financial status changes. Your job situation changes.

It affects your self-worth. Your self-esteem. Your confidence. Your rhythms. The way you breathe. Your mentality. Your brain function. (Ever heard the term "Widow Brain? If you don't know what that is, consider yourself lucky.") Your physical body.

Your hobbies and interests. Your sense of security. Your sense of humor.
Your sense of womanhood or manhood.

EVERY. SINGLE. THING. CHANGES.

You are handed a new life that you never asked for
and that you don't particularly want. It is the hardest, most
gut-wrenching, horrific, life-altering of things to live with."

I have to try hard to remember this:

It's hard when you miss people, but you know,
if you miss them, it means you were lucky.

It means you had someone special in your life, someone worth missing.

I am thankful that I had someone to love as much as I did.

~

November 24

First Thanksgiving without him. Dinner at Michelle's. Something doesn't
feel right. Boo Hoo!

~

November 30

Reminiscing. 28 years ago, today when Beecher and I met, 11-30-88.

~

December 4

Elks Lodge had a memorial for all the departed Elks this year. It was a nice ceremony but it was hard seeing Beecher's picture on the wall with the words –" Departed Brother." Many times, I've been in the Lodge, and I've seen all the pictures of all the Exalted Rulers and the ones with the black ribbon on them that represented a Departed Brother. Now seeing that black ribbon on his picture seems so surreal.

December 5

I contacted Pash again about the RJ article and she said it keeps getting pushed back by the editor and the holidays are a tricky time of year. She said she knows it will eventually run. Once it does run, she will get me a hard copy as well.

December 7

Beecher was laid to rest today as he journeyed back home on Dec. 7, 2016, on the 75th Anniversary of the Pearl Harbor attack.

As Beecher was a Veteran, we "Honored his Spirit" at the VA Memorial and Burial Cemetery "Going Home" ceremony. More beautiful music was played and sung by our dear friend, Stephanie. I was honored to have the Minister that had married us in 1991 and then at our first vow renewal in 1995 administer the program and do the Gravesite Dedication. As is the custom for Vets, Beecher received full Navy Honors Taps and a Flag Ceremony. I was presented with the American Flag for his service in the Navy Seabees. The ceremony in the Chapel ended with the song "Silver Thunderbird" by Marc Cohn. It was one of Beecher's favorite songs by Marc, as it talked about when he died, he wanted to go down in a Silver Thunderbird. You have to listen to the song to understand the meaning. (My daughter Amy had been fortunate to find two model Silver Thunderbirds, one that now rests on the top of his wooden, chrome plated urn that sits on top of my fireplace with some of his ashes. There is also another one in his grave with his ashes). Amy got up and said a few words, saying how grateful she was to have had Beecher as a stepfather. She said his influence had made her a stronger person and how glad I had brought him into our lives. A special thanks goes to everyone who attended and to those who sent flowers and donations in lieu of flowers to theAFTD.org in honor of Beecher.

~

December 15

I took a trip to Cedar City, UT with Amy. Enjoyed four days of doing nothing but relaxing.

~

December 25, Christmas Day

Dinner at my grandson Justin's house. I was able to buy gifts for everyone this year. First time in many years. So sad without Beech. Miss him so much.

~

December 31, 2016

The year is over and my husband is gone. I went to our friends Dave and Anita's to celebrate New Year's with them and some of their friends. Left twenty minutes before New Year's. Wanted to be alone. (Amy had gone with the WolfCreek band to Surprise, AZ to ring in the New Year).

Being a caregiver for so long you never actually forget how difficult it is to live the journey and unless you live the journey you don't know what an emotional roller coaster it is. As the end gets near, you some-times pray to God to let it be over soon and sometimes you feel selfish for saying that. There are days you think it's over and then it's not and you feel let down. You just want it to be over for them as well as you. There is a sadness in that all that you have been through is soon coming to an end. There is a reality and an emptiness that I am no longer a care-giver, so who am I now? I'm no longer a wife, I'm a widow. I'd rather say I'm single or divorced than say "widow." If I ever get married again, am I no longer a widow? Or do I take on the new title as "wife" again even though I was left a widow? And if I marry again and lose another husband, am I a widow twice removed? All these questions, I ask myself. Was my husband afraid to leave this world? Did Beecher hang on so long because he was afraid I couldn't survive without him or because he still needed me and he knew I needed him? I often wonder if I could have done better. I often felt guilty because of all the times I yelled at him. Would he have yelled at me if the roles had been reversed? He never complained, except in the beginning and then later it didn't faze him: he just accepted it, or I quit yelling. I kept it in and screamed inside at myself. I wish I knew what I know now, but it's always easier to reflect back in time than when you're living it. I just did my best that I could do, and I am learning to forgive myself. My counselor once told me that FTD patients live in the moment and don't think about the past or future.

I'm learning that grief is not about the person that died, but it's about us and how we feel about our life now and that we are no longer a care-giver for someone we cared so deeply for. It's about rebuilding and facing a new life now that a huge part of life is missing. I'm learning that grief is something you can't push through. You have to absorb it, adjust to it and accept it and that it's not something you just all of a sudden complete. Instead, you just endure it, and you never finish it. You have to alter yourself and find a new way of seeing and becoming a new defini-tion of who you are - your new self. We have to find ourselves because we disappeared along with our loved one. I feel because I had devoted so much time to being a caregiver, that I no longer have a purpose in life. I feel empty like there is something more I should be doing.

Trying to create new routines is hard because I had developed a purpose in life taking care of him and now there is none unless I create new ones. I'm already thinking of going back to playing tennis, learning pickle ball, play a little golf, start walking every day, and getting back to my dance classes, but I seem to keep making excuses for not getting started. I'm also thinking of taking ballroom dance lessons or piano lessons like I always wanted to. All it requires is putting one foot in front of the other. Why is that so hard? It takes so much effort and I guess I'm not quite ready for it. Some days I feel like I am falling apart. I cry when I hear our favorite songs. I cry when I look at his many pictures, I have all over the house or in the endless albums I have made for years. But it is getting better and I find myself sometimes smiling when I see a picture of him and his sense of humor shows through. But finally, FINALLY, I am almost done with my last task to honor him and I am already feeling better. I feel my new life is just around the corner.

As I wrap up this book, please understand that as much as I griped and complained, I **never** did not love my husband. He was the best thing that ever happened to me and I will never regret any part of my life with him. Many of you reading this book that have a loved one with FTD may not experience the same issues I did. Your journey may be longer or shorter. To those who aren't familiar with this disease, I ask you to learn about it and spread the word to your family and friends. You never know when that thief may come in the middle of the night and steal your loved one's brain and your heart and soul. Your knowledge may help someone else who is suffering from a misdiagnosed condition and you can help them get an earlier diagnosis. I pray that a cure with come soon so no one else has to experience the journey and grief that we went through. God Bless you all.

Grief never ends, but it changes
It's a passage, not a place to stay
Grief is not a sign of weakness,
Not a lack of faith.
It is the price of love.

Author Unknown

CHAPTER 7

LETTING GO & MOVING FORWARD

LIFE AFTER BEECH GOES ON

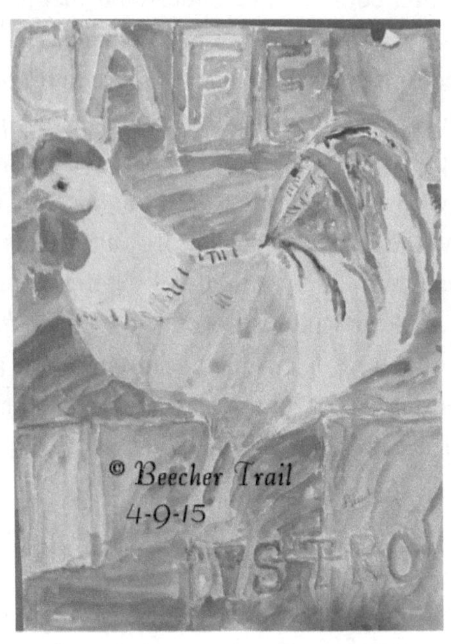

"Year of the Rooster"
Watercolor by Beecher Trail
"The Rooster represents the symbol of a rising sun and a new day"

~LETTING GO & MOVING FORWARD (TRYING TO)~: RECOVERY OF GETTING OVER THE LOSS!

January 1

Stayed up till midnight since I stayed so late at Dave and Anita's. First time in a long time. Beecher and I hadn't stayed up in years. We usually stayed home to avoid the traffic.

This year will be my recovery of getting over the loss of my husband and trying to deal with my life "after Beech." Discovering what the rest of my life will be life. Where do I go from here? What has God planned for me? Been getting a lot of rest and taking care of myself.

First thing on agenda; doctor appts, dental, vision, and blood work.

Second thing; get things fixed on car; tires rotated, oil change, alignment, brakes, and paint hood of car that I've put off for a year. (I was afraid to be without a car for two days).

Third thing; declutter my house, top to bottom, including my car and garage. Get my office in order, especially.

Hope to do some traveling, get my passport renewed, and start back to my exercise class and watercolor class. Lunch with old and new friends that I've missed seeing the last few years. Time to move forward and see what life has in store for me.

Letting go of fear. In our Firewalk classes which were Goal Setting Seminars and walking over hot coals, we used to jokingly say that the word FEAR meant Forget Everything And Run, but what it really meant is False Evidence Appearing Real. Our motto was:

> *When I dare to be powerful –*
> *To use my strength in the*
> *Service of my vision,*
> *Then it becomes less*
> *And less*
> *Important whether I am afraid.*

Sometimes you just have to turn the page to realize there is more to your book of life than the page you are stuck on. I have been stuck on this page for quite a while and it's time to remember what we taught and stop being afraid to move on. It's fear that keeps us stuck.

At some point you just have to let go of what you thought should happen and live in what is happening.

And then it happens,
One day you wake up and you're in this place
You're in this place where everything feels right.
Your heart is calm.
Your soul is lit.
Your thoughts are positive.
Your vision is clear.
You're at peace, at peace with
Where you've been, at peace
With what you've been through
And at peace with where you're headed.
(Credit to the Mind Journal)

One of the happiest moments in life is when you find the courage to let go of what you can't change. As the Serenity Prayer from NA says:

God grant me
The Serenity to accept the things I cannot change
Courage to change the things I can and
Wisdom to know the difference.
(Credit to Alcoholics Anonymous)

I'm hoping that I find that moment soon, so I can be at peace with where I'm headed.

That's all!

Well, maybe one more thing or two! I just realized that writing a book takes a long time even when you have a journal to start with. There is so much more information to put in it! As I put the finishing touches on getting this book ready for publication, I have shed many tears as I read and re-read the book numerous times, adding, deleting, spell checking and making sure I hadn't left out anything important. I hadn't read my journal since Beecher passed away and I forgot how difficult it was for both him and me as his wife and caregiver for over 28 years. As I read through all my daily thoughts, worries and daily experiences day after day, it's a wonder how I made it through. At the time it's all happening you just learn to deal with it, but after it's over it seems impossible to have survived this journey. I remember thinking at the time that I would never get through it, but now my life without him is the hardest and most difficult thing of all. It's weird how your prospective can change that quickly. I hope I can live the best life the way he would have wanted me to and the way I know he would have if the roles had been reversed. This hellish journey will always make me emotional and will most likely make me cry every time I read this book, or portions of it, but it will also bring me many good memories that will make me laugh. Those memories will be embedded in my mind forever. His illness created an everlasting bond that will last for eternity. I'm thankful that he chose me as his soul mate. I know that someday we will be together again. "Dantatsu!" He was the best of the best!

February 7

Today I got a call from Nicole Wolf who is the Director of Marketing for the Brain Center in Las Vegas. She told me that I had been chosen to be interviewed for the Keep Memory Alive 21st Annual Power of Love Gala event at the MGM Grand Garden Arena. This year, Keep Memory Alive is paying a special tribute to caregivers who have gone above and beyond to care for loved ones suffering from these devastating diseases and I am one of them. I will be highlighted in a special video tribute along with three other caregivers. I am honored to be part of this.

Siegfried of Siegfried and Roy will be honored with the Caregiver Award. Following Roy's accident that left him with physical limitations,

Siegfried provided around the clock care to his best friend for almost fifteen years. This is the first year the award will be given and will become an annual tradition. In addition, Andre Agassi will be awarded the Community Leadership Award for his philanthropic achievements for the great state of Nevada. Keep Memory Alive mission is to provide enhanced treatment and ultimately cures for patients and their families suffering from neurocognitive disorders, including FTD and raises awareness and funds in support of the Cleveland Clinic Lou Ruvo Center for Brain Health.

The Power of Love Gala started as a celebration of life in 1996 when Keep Memory Alive founder, Larry Ruvo, had a dinner with some friends to celebrate his late father, Lou Ruvo, who passed away from Alzheimer's disease. Over the dinner, Larry received donations in the amount of $30,000 from his friends to put towards research. This donation eventually led to bringing the esteemed Cleveland Clinic to Las Vegas and funded the Cleveland Clinic Lou Ruvo Center for Brain Health. Since 1996, Keep Memory Alive has served as the sole fundraising arm for the Cleveland Clinic Lou Ruvo Center for Brain Health.

In the past two decades, the Power of Love Gala, a spectacular evening dedicated to fighting the ravages of Alzheimer's disease and other neurocognitive disorders, has blossomed into a celebration known for partnering with some of the most celebrated chefs and entertainers in the industry for an evening of philanthropy, while raising crucial awareness and funds for Keep Memory Alive in support of the Clinic.

February 15

Nicole texted me that her video crew from Cleveland is coming out to Vegas the week of March 20 and they would love to film me for the Power of Love Gala. We set the date for March 20 to film me at my home.

~

March 14

Nicole texted me again with information on how to prepare for the interview. In addition, she wanted me to have some of Beecher's artwork handy as they wanted to film that. Some of the questions she would ask me included:

1. When did you first realize you'd become a caregiver for your husband?
2. What does being a caregiver involve?
3. Tell us what it's like: difficult, and why? Filled with humor sometimes and why?
4. Who was there to support me? Tell them about the role of friend and family.
5. How did Cleveland Clinic help?
6. How has life changed since his passing and you're no longer a full-time caregiver?

In answer to Question #1

I first realized I was becoming a caregiver in May 2013 when my husband was diagnosed with PPA and was told that he wasn't going to get better, and that PPA was most likely caused by FTD.

Question #2

Being a caregiver involves a lot of patience, learning to understand the illness, being prepared for changes, such as personality changes, social demeanor, intimacy issues, accepting new challenges every day, handling comments of other people in public, learning how to become a mother to a 6'2", 58-year-old man baby. It involves trying not to beat yourself up every time you act mean or insensitive to him. Watching after him every minute of the day and night as you try and keep him safe.

Learning to deal with grief and saying I'm sorry over and over and over. Dealing with his obsessive behaviors, incontinence issues, cleaning up after him in the men's public restrooms, safety issues, falls, walking off in a store, guilty for putting him in a home.

Question #3

Being a caregiver was the most difficult role I've ever had in my life! In the beginning I was angry at him and at God and at life itself. I felt sorry for myself that I had been given this burden. No one can prepare you for the devastation of seeing your loved one become a person you no longer know. One that you can no longer communicate with. No hopes and dreams for the future. Accepting the disease as terminal. Since I'm 8 years older, I always thought he would take care of me in my old age. He always said he would go before me. We had a saying that he would get older but he would never grow up because he was such a kid at heart, and I would say "I've spent my whole life raising kids, but I'll spend the rest of my life raising him." How little did I know that statement would come true. Watching him become more and more childlike every day instead of growing old with me.

The car accidents and dealing with insurance companies and lawyers. Our social life changed, and most of his friends or couples became distant. I think they didn't know how to handle it. My biggest challenges were finding resources to help ease the burden, which took many hours of the day, i.e. (learning about and applying for grants, unemployment for him, VA benefits and VA Pension so I could put him in a home, seeking an attorney regarding wills & trusts, life insurance, dealing with a lawsuit from an accident he had, learning to sell on e-bay and Craigslist to ease some financial burdens, searching for group homes etc. and all the while doing the daily shopping, finances, doctors visit for him and myself and on and on.) It seemed like it never ended. Never ending paperwork. Asking for help. Staying strong for my daughters.

I think I survived because of some of the wonderful memories he gave us in spite of the illness. Yes, sometimes he gave us many memories of some of the funny things he did, or the expressions on his face told us he was still in there somewhere. i.e. (the day at the VA with the man whose butt crack was showing), the day my friend went with me to visit him and took the bad jelly beans, the day he wiped his mouth with a napkin to get a kiss, the day he flipped his middle finger at his high school friend because he couldn't get his fingers made into the I love you sign anymore. The expressions on his face were priceless!

Question # 4

The people that supported me most were: My two daughters mostly, my brothers and sisters here locally and in California, and good close friends of mine. Adult day care (feeling relief that I had eight hours one day a week to myself), Visiting Angels, one in particular who became Franny the Nanny. She was truly an Angel (gave me respite time four days a week for four hours, cleaned my home, cooked for us, played Scrabble with my husband.) It gave me time to go shopping or just get out of the house for a few hours. Friends from the club where we took watercolor lessons and dance classes. Our teachers were so sweet and understanding of his condition and many became very good friends.

Question #5

Cleveland Clinic helped me in many ways. Social workers, the support group with Lisa Radin, financial support and the genuine caring of the doctors and nurses who made me feel that I wasn't alone. Dr. Léger for his kindness and deep empathy who helped me each step of the way to understand the illness.

Question #6

Since my husband passed and I'm no longer a caregiver, I feel like an enormous burden has been lifted off my chest, but in some ways, I still feel a need to take care of someone but no longer want the burden. I feel like something is missing. The habits of getting up and taking care of him or to go to the home to visit him, take him to the doctor, or take him a milkshake. As hard as it was, I feel empty inside; like he should still be here and I should still be taking care of him. My life is just now starting to move forward after five months of his passing. I'm starting to get back to my watercolor classes and dance classes. Knowing that I can go where I want anytime, anywhere, eat when I want, watch TV when I want, sleep when I want and yet at times, wishing I still had him here to do all those things with him. It's very lonely at this stage. I'm learning to take care of myself, my health, my teeth, my car; things that I neglected because I was busy taking care of him. Getting back in touch with old friends that I hadn't had time for. Working on my journal that I started four years ago, that I hope to publish someday. Learning to live alone for the first time in my life.

~

March 20

The video crew from Cleveland Clinic in Ohio arrived on time and the interview went very well. Nicole and the crew, Dave, Mike and Val were very nice and showed a lot of compassion as I told my story. They filmed for over an hour. During some of my emotional times, I often saw tears in their eyes and I knew they had been moved by my honesty.

One of the guys gave me a big hug when it was over and confided in me that he had a son with a rare disease so he knew what I was going through and I felt a connection with him. As they were leaving my home a big asphalt company truck came down the street and I pointed out that that was what Beecher did for a living.

I said, "I think Beecher is watching over me and wants to know what I'm doing with three guys in the house."

They all got a laugh out of that. The next day I got a text from Nicole to thank me for welcoming them into my home and sharing my story with them.

She said I was honest, open and candid with them and it was exactly the type of inside look into life as a caregiver that she was hoping to hear. She hopes it will reassure other caregivers they're not alone and that resources are available to help and perhaps inspire Gala attendees to step up and give.

She thanked me for my hospitality and that it was a delight to meet me and get to know Beecher through my loving stories.

Nicole and all the guys gave me great big hugs when they left. I informed them that we all needed twelve hugs a day for maintenance and to always hug heart to heart. I had sent a text to the guys to thank them and she had read the text and said they were very touched and sent back lots of hugs; heart to heart, of course.

April 18

I got the confirmation from MacKenzie informing me we are scheduled to film with Katie Boer of KLAS-CBS from Channel 8 tomorrow the 19th at my home to do the story on Beecher and said the segment will run the week of the Power of Love Gala on April 27.

Afterward, they will head to the Brain Center to film with Dr. Léger. I sent quite a few photos and videos of Beecher to use for the episode. Evidently, Pash from the RJ no longer works there and Katie is taking over the segment and wants to televise it on Channel 8 instead of the article in the RJ that was scheduled to run last year.

April 19

Katie Boer and her camera crew came to my home to do the interview and filming and it went very well. Afterwards, Katie requested some photos and videos I have of Beecher which they wanted to use in the episode on Ch. 8.

April 21

Katie contacted me by email and explained how the breakdown of how the stories would go. She plans to split it into 2 stories as such:

Introduction of me and Beecher, getting the diagnosis, the struggles, what it was like becoming a caregiver, ending on me being honored at the Power of Love Gala. Also, some added explanations from Dr. Léger.

More on Beecher's experience, about him becoming a talented water color artist, more in-depth explanation from Dr. Léger about what specifically was happening in Beecher's brain. And the efforts that are being done in terms of research and clinical trials.

The interview that I did for Channel 8 News aired in two parts on April 25 and 26 and also ran online at LasVegasNow.com. The first part was titled "Beecher the Preacher" and the second part was titled "Beecher the Painter." Katie Boer, the reporter did an excellent job of putting it together and it was nice that it aired the same week of the Power of Love Gala at the MGM. In addition to that a CBS affiliate station picked up the story in Myrtle Beach, South Carolina so my story is officially nation-wide! Hoping that other affiliates picked it up as we need to raise more awareness about FTD. Also, CNN Newspath and CBS has requested the two stories so they would be aired in full, or a shorter summary in other cities across the country as well.

This is so amazing! The more people that see it, the more people will learn about FTD and understand it and many will get an earlier diagnosis. Already my daughter's friend saw it on Facebook and told my daughter that her husband might have it. They had been wondering what was wrong with him and after watching the videos they felt that that's what it was. My daughter encouraged her to make an appointment at the Brain Center. I was honored to do the interview as I know my husband would have done the same. He always believed in making a difference and his favorite saying by Gandhi was "You must be the change you wish to see in the world." I'm proud to be able to carry on his message and to inspire and make a difference in other people's lives. It feels good to be able to do something in Beecher's name after he's gone. I'm sure he is looking down on me and smiling.

After it aired, my youngest daughter Amy sent me this wonderful note:

Mommy, I commend you for giving such an honest, tearful and powerful representation of his struggles as well as the care giving aspect of this disease. The Channel 8 News did such a great job of putting it all together to tell a painful yet beautiful summary of his illness. We had to see the beauty in even the hardest moments. His paintings were proof of that and gifts that will live on forever. As well as the memories and the laughs we shared even in some of the toughest moments we all had to endure. I am crying my eyes out finally getting to watch these segments. It hurts to re-live these moments, but I know daddy would want us to do what we can to help raise awareness so they can find a cure. I am SO happy to know they will be honoring you at the Power of Love Gala event! You deserve it and I know you will keep doing good things with the responsibilities he left you to help make a difference like he always strived to do. Mommy, you are the true Rockstar of the family. I am so proud of you and honored to be your daughter! Thank you for setting an example for us all. I love you more than words can possibly say!

Note: (The Caregiver video for the Power of Love Gala that was held at the MGM Grand Arena was aired on April 27, 2017 and included my interview.)

~

July 5

Danielle Kemeny from the Cleveland Clinic Brain Health Donation Program called me to tell me she is sending a preliminary report to me within a week in regards to Beecher's brain donation. The lab wants to do a staining of his brain as they think it's a real interesting case and "not common." It will take an additional month or two for the full report as they have to order a staining kit. The investigator will be available if I want to talk to him or if I have any questions.

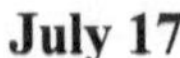

July 17

I received the brain autopsy report today. It's been almost nine months. It has taken a lot longer than originally anticipated due to the fact that they have been back logged. I don't know if that's good or bad. Either too many people dying from this disease or more people choosing to do the brain donation. I prefer to think it's the latter. They were able to get the staining kit earlier than they thought and they were able to speed up the process. The findings are as follows:

My husband was diagnosed with frontotemporal dementia, primary progressive aphasia with Corticobasal syndrome subtype. The findings at autopsy confirmed this <u>clinical diagnosis.</u> They observed changes in the brain that were consistent with a diagnosis of Corticobasal Degeneration. Specifically, they observed the characteristics of changes in the brain including a predominant 4-repeat TAU deposition throughout the brain.

August 4

I talked to the investigator today regarding the pathology report since I was somewhat confused about the results. He explained to me the following:

1. FTD umbrella includes CBS
2. CBS was the most common change throughout the pathology report.
3. Language problems is usually the first symptom of CBS
4. Problems with motor skills typically causes disease to go faster.
5. There are two types of TAU, 3 –repeat and 4-repeat.
   Beecher's was predominately 4-repeat TAU indicating CBS.

6. There were no signs of traumatic changes in the brain that would indicate head trauma had caused CBS

7. Anesthesia (he had had a lot) could cause him struggling to recover as fast but there was no indication of cause—maybe not enough of research at this time.

8. The staining kit helped determine the TAU pathology to confirm it as CBS.

9. The most important factor is: CBS typically does not run, in families. This is important to his sisters, nieces, nephews and down the genetic line. They can be assured that they will less likely inherit CBS. I was happy to be able to report this finding to his sisters and family. This was a real blessing, and I'm glad that I had his brain donated.

To sum it up, CBS – Corticobasal Degeneration was the Neuropathological finding. And the clinical diagnosis was FTD and PPA with Corticobasal Syndrome subtype. What I found interesting was that the investigator was not aware of the clinical findings from the doctors until after the autopsy. The reason for this is so they don't assume any past results from the doctors and they want to base the autopsy on their findings only.

Somewhere on Facebook someone posted this awhile back and there is no name as to who wrote it, but I feel it needs to be in my book, so here it is:

A thief crept into my home one night,
but how he came in
and how he left
is still not answered quite right.

Diamonds and pearls were not the goal,
gold and coins lay untouched,
and TV's and stereos
all kept their dust.

What he took was much more precious
than any of these, and
even worse was
what he left with me.

This thief, this devil,
this blight unknown,
he stole my heart
and very soul.

In he came,
with no backward glance
and took the mind
of my very best friend.

Overnight it seemed, all I had known
was now replaced with the unknown
and someone unfamiliar
in my loved one's place.

What right?
I thought
and "just you wait."
But it was too late,

For already he had
escaped from my estate.
Now what? Which way do I turn?
How can I fix this damage he's done?

I already knew
the answer was mute,
not enough research,
no good news.

Here I sit alone
with hopes and prayers,
chatting with others
who have suffered the same insane thievery?

Hope against hope
that he can be caught or stopped
and that ways will be found
to undo his foul harm.

Until then my friends,
beware the thief,
lock your doors,
and secure the windows.

Never take those you love
for granted, for you cannot know how
or when this thief may come in,
and prey upon your life's best friend.

Just when I was typing the last words in my book, a good friend of ours, Lynn sent me a message telling me the following words had popped up on her Facebook page from several years ago, when her mother passed away. I'm not sure if these were Beecher's words or someone else but these are the words Beecher sent to her to comfort her:

Every life has a beginning and an end. However, when someone we love a great deal reaches the end of their life, we may have a very hard time accepting their sudden, final absence. Our grief may be so powerful that we fear it will completely overwhelm us – but it will not. Our sorrow may hurt more than anything we can remember, but it will pass. We need not run from the emotions that may arise from the death of a loved one. Death and grieving are part of the fullness of living "life on life's terms." By allowing ourselves the freedom to experience these feelings, we partake more deeply of both our recovery and our human nature. Sometimes the reality of another's death makes our own mortality that much more pronounced. We reevaluate our priorities, appreciating the loved ones still with us all the more. Our life, and our life with them, will not go on forever. We want to make the most of what's important while it lasts. We might find that the death of someone we love helps strengthen our conscious contact with our Higher Power. If we remember that we can always turn to that source of strength when we are troubled, we will be able to stay focused on it no matter what may be going on around us.

CONTRIBUTORS

Foreword

Dr. Gabriel Léger, Neurologist- Past Director of the Frontotemporal and Young-onset Dementias Program at Cleveland Clinic Lou Ruvo Center for Brain Health in Las Vegas, Nevada and currently a Neurology Specialist in San Diego, California at the University of California San Diego Health.

Preface

Lisa Radin- Former Caregiver and co-author of "What If Its Not Alzheimer's? A Caregivers Guide to Dementia," Support-group Facilitator and has been involved in planning and coordinating FTD Caregiver Conferences.

ABOUT THE AUTHOR

Nancy Trail provided complete care for her husband, Beecher for four years after he was diagnosed with Progressive Primary Aphasia (PPA) with Corticobasal syndrome (CBS) and Frontotemporal Degeneration (FTD). Prior to her commitment to taking care of him with this devastating disease, she was a loving and devoted wife and is the mother of three, grandmother of seven and great grandmother of six. Nancy spent most of her career as a Comptroller for a Title Insurance Company, a Sales Rep in several industries, an Aesthetician, a motivational speaker with their Trails of Fire business and the creator of a Fitness Camp for Ladies Only, called Heart, Body & Soul. She spent many weekends for several years assisting Rapport Leadership International volunteering as a staff member at their weekend personal growth seminars. She currently resides in the Las Vegas area.

TIPS FOR CAREGIVERS

Legal Affairs

- Choose a Power of Attorney for Health Care and Financial Decisions
- Create a Living Will and Trust

Community Resources

- Check out the Adult Day Care Centers in your area well in advance.
- Check out different types of Memory Care facilities in your area. They may vary from city to city.

Support Groups

- Join a support group for yourself. If none are in your area, create one. You will be helping yourself as well as others.
- Visiting Angels or other similar agencies in your area. If you're loved one is a VET, contact your local VA.

Hospice

- Find out where the nearest one is in your area. Be prepared ahead of time.

Coping with Memory Loss

- Keep a list of all appointments for your loved one as well as yourself, post phone numbers in large print, including emergency numbers and your address in case your loved one is home alone and make sure they know where the numbers are posted. Set up automatic bill pay with your bank. It makes it one less thing to remember to do.

Nursing Home and Assisted Living

- Visit nearby nursing homes and assisted living facilities well in advance so you can be prepared for the costs and availability when the time comes. It can sneak up on you.

Websites

- Keep a list of the pertinent websites that you refer to often and so you can have the list handy when others want more information about the illness. Let them do the reading, you have enough on your hands, and sometimes they need to read it themselves to completely understand this disease. Many people may not believe what you are going through. Only others that are experiencing the same disease will truly understand and have empathy for you. Many people will have "sympathy" for you but the ones who have walked in your shoes and have gone through the same thing will be the ones who have "empathy" for you. This is the difference in sympathy and empathy.

Do Not Contact for Caregiver's List Registration

- As I mentioned in Chapter 3, 2013, I stated that I contacted PCH (Publisher's Clearing House) in regards to continued use by my husband with his debit card. They put a block on his account and closed it so he could not order any more items and they put "opted out" due to dementia. It may take up to 4-8 weeks for the block to go into effect. In addition, they removed him from the general mailing list and credited back his debit card as well. Their number is 1-800-459-4724. PHC also referred me to contact www.dmachoice.org which is the Direct Marketing Association to have him removed from all other general Direct mailings. Once you notify them, they will email you and ask you to confirm your registration for the Do Not Contact for Caregiver's List Registration and the link to confirm the activation and verification. After doing so, I never had any further problems.

RESOURCES

Books

Radin, Lisa & Gary *"What If It's Not Alzheimer's? A Caregiver's Guide to Dementia,"* Prometheus Books, 3rd Edition, 2014

Soloway, Elaine, *"Green Nails and other Acts of Rebellion,"* Life After Loss, She Writes Press, 2014

Nelson, Nancy *"Blue. River. Apple."* An exploration of Alzheimer's through Poetry, 2014

Mautner Ph.D., Raeleen D'Agostino, *"Lemons into Limoncello,"* From Loss to Personal Renaissance with the Zest of Italy, Health Communications, Inc., 2013

Rasmussen, Christina, *"Second Firsts"* Live, Laugh and Love Again" Hay House, Inc. 2013

Sandberg, Sheryl & Grant, Adam, *Option B, Facing Adversity, Building Resilience, and Finding Joy,* Borzoi, 2017

Colgrove, Ph.D., Melba, *"How to Survive the Loss of a Love,"* Bantam Books, 1976

Bennett, Michael Gordon, *"Rusty's War: A Battle of the Mind,"* Bennett Global Entertainment, 2017

"Watercolors by Beecher Trail 2013-2016" May be purchased directly from Nancy Trail.
You can email her at crystalgal@cox.net.

All proceeds will go to The Association for Frontotemporal Degeneration (FTD)

Magazine

Cleveland Clinic Lou Ruvo Center for Brain Health, *"New Thinking, about Thinking" a Semi-Annual Publication.* Keepmemoryalive.org and clevelandclinic.org/brainhealth

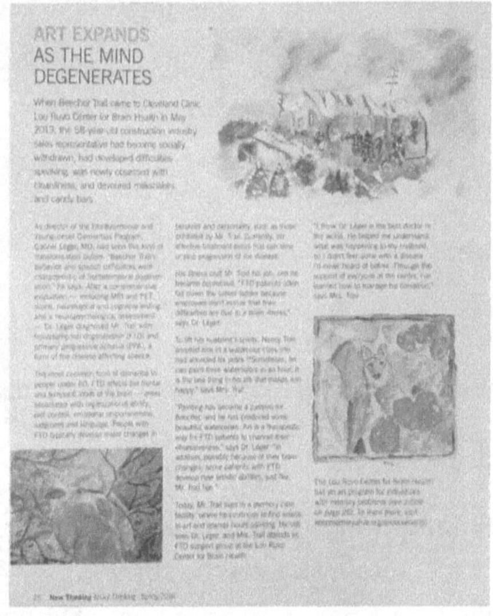

Booklets

The Association for Frontotemporal Degeneration (AFTD), *"The Doctor Thinks It's FTD, Now What?" A guide for Managing a New Diagnosis,* www.theaftd.org *info @theaftd.org, 2013

"Understanding the Genetics of FTD," A Guide for Patients and Their Families. University of Pennsylvania Center for Neurodegenerative Disease Research, Penn Medicine 2012

Websites

The Association for Frontotemporal Degeneration (FTD): www.theaftd.org

Alzheimer's: https://alz.org

Visiting Angels –Las Vegas, Nevada 702-562-3322 www.visitingangels.com

Vet Angels -1-800-319-1117 www.vetangels.org

Helping Hands – Las Vegas, Nevada 702-633-7264 http://hhvv.org

Nathan Adelson Hospice: www.nah.org

Videos and YouTube:

"Power of Love" – Celebrating Caregivers http://www.keepmemoryalive.org/caregivers/patient_caregiver_services/education

YouTube of Beecher and Nancy with Dr. Léger from Lunch and Learn at the Lou Ruvo Brain Center on October 5, 2016 https://www.youtube.com/Keep-memory-alive-FTD-observations

"Beecher the Preacher" - First segment aired April 25, 2017
http://www.8newsnow.com/news/lesser-known-dementia-ftd-robs-people-of-language-skills/699422180

"Beecher the Painter" - Second segment aired April 26, 2017
http://www.8newsnow.com/news/mans-spiral-into-dementia-revealed-artistic-ability/699891766

"FTD Awareness " and "Coping with Creativity" – Ch. 5 – Fox 5 Special Reports with anchor John Huck – November 25, 26 and 27, 2019
"FTD Awareness –"Losing Stephanie – Las Vegas Woman Suffers from Rare Form of Dementia" November 25, 2019 (Beecher is also included in this)
https://facebook.com/watch/?v=2371125289664885

"Coping Through Creativity—Type of dementia seen in Las Vegas patients inspires art in some" November 27, 2019 Special Report: Type of Dementia.
https://www.fox5vegas.com/2019/11/27/special-report-type-dementia-seen-las-vegas-patients-inspire-art-some

Several people responded after watching Coping Through Creativity:

"I started sobbing when I saw the deceased man's watercolors that he suddenly took up after this disease. How beautiful that he could leave behind such beauty. Such a sad way to lose someone. Brain disease is cruel."

"That gentleman's water color paintings were amazing!!"

∼

To be a more effective well-informed caregiver, visit
www.keepmemoryalive.org and select "patient and family services."

Brain Donation Programs:
Contact Danielle Kemeny @Cleveland Clinic in Cleveland, Ohio 216-445-7110 or KemenyD@ccf.org as of this writing.

There is also another brain support facility in California called Brain Support Network. As of this writing, Robin Riddle is the contact person at 650-814-0848 orwww.brainsupportnetwork.org

BIBLIOGRAPHY

"A Fallen Limb poem" pg. 126 Author Unknown
"Grief Never Ends quote" pg. 131 Author Unknown
"A Thief poem" pg. 139 Author Unknown

ACKNOWLEDGMENTS

I couldn't have written this book without the help of the many people in my life. First and foremost, I want to thank my beautiful loving daughters, Michelle and Amy for their undying love for me and for Beecher. Although, he was not their real father, they loved him as if he were and he was always there for them, not because he had to be, but because he wanted to be. My daughters kept me grounded at times when I thought I would lose it and they encouraged me to be strong. They gave me the strength and courage to get through each day. I love and thank you both for being by my side and I'm so grateful you were with me and him right through to the end as he passed from this life to the next. I love you more than words can say.

Heartfelt thanks to my sisters, Linda and Patti and my brothers, Donny and Ricky who were never more than a phone call away and helped me financially and emotionally during the toughest times. Patti often picked us up and took us to lunch and the movies, after stopping at the 99 Cent store so he could have candy during the movies. You are all much appreciated!

Special thanks to my longtime dearest friend, Sandy Coffman who was always there for moral support and love. Also, to my dear friend Belinda Enger, whom I met in watercolor class who was also dealing with her husband's health issue at the same time. We were always there for each other as we dealt with different issues. She was my shoulder to cry on many times and vice versa as we both knew what each other was going through. She visited Beecher with me many times and she always managed to get him to get all us to laugh. Also, my girlfriends from high school whom I met with monthly for lunch that gave me back some of my sanity.

Thanks to Sylvia Bachiochi (who is now deceased), our watercolor teacher who had a heart of gold and patience and took the time to assist Beecher in class so I could paint without too much interruption.

Thanks, and gratitude to Frances Sweetman, our Visiting Angel, who blessed our home with her love and compassion as she attended to Beecher, fixing meals, cleaning my home and giving me respite time so I could attend to the many tasks I had to take care of on a daily basis. She often sat with Beecher playing checkers, and Scrabble and encouraged him to read from his Narcotics Anonymous (herein referred to as NA) book each time she visited. She went above and beyond, and I appreciate her enormously for her devotion to us. She has become a very special friend.

A huge thanks to Lisa Radin whom I was so lucky to have as my mentor and guide to help me through this journey. How blessed I was to live in Las Vegas and be a part of her support group. Her book, "What if It's Not Alzheimer's? A Caregiver's Guide to Dementia" gave me so much knowledge and inspiration for writing this book. Being in her support group and sharing with others helped me understand that I was not alone. She was always a phone call away if I needed to vent.

Thanks to Dr. Gabriel Léger, Beecher's Neurologist, whose wisdom, knowledge, experience in FTD, and his loving nature and compassion made our journey bearable. His knowledge of FTD and his desire to find a cure is remarkable. Thank you, Dr. Léger for always returning my calls within a short time, and for receiving my non-emergency questions through My Chart. And thank you to his nurse Nancy, who often replied the same day.

Thanks to Dr. Dylan Wint, Beecher's Psychiatrist, who gave me and Beecher comfort when the issue of attempted suicide was discussed. I especially appreciated his words of empathy when he said to me "I don't know how people deal with this disease. It is so heartbreaking. You're taking care of a 6'2" 5-year-old." He understood so well what I was going through.

Thanks to Jenna Clifford, my therapist at Lou Ruvo, who helped guide me through the many frustrations, anxiety, guilt and feelings of grief and loss. Even though she was not counseling me at the end of his life, she helped me understand and deal with the loss as I traveled through the journey.

Thanks to the Elks Lodge #1468 for their love and support for helping me out financially in times of need, for use of the Lodge for Beecher's Benefit to raise money, and for use of the Lodge for his Celebration of Life. His many Elks Brothers and Sisters loved him and often took the time to take us to lunch and check on us.

A big thanks to Linda Stone from Vetangels.org who took the time to explain to me how to file a claim for Aid & Attendance with the VA. She guided me through each step of the way to help me apply in a timely manner and she was always a phone call away. She asked for nothing in return, donations only if you have it. No pressure. Another Angel for sure!

Thanks to the VA Southwest Primary Care Clinic with special thanks to the social worker, Jennifer Daley Dawson, for helping me secure Beecher's Respite Care and setting up Visiting Angels. Thanks to nurse, Jacqueline who helped me with the Hospice Eligibility and was always there to assist me with any situation that arose in regards to Beecher's health and for always returning my calls in a timely manner. You made my journey easier.

And to all the doctors at the VA, too many to list, who were involved in his care (the primary doctors, the mental health doctor, the med doctor, the other nurses and to the Rehab Center doctors at the Veterans Benefit Administration in regards to obtaining compression socks and wheelchairs.)

Thanks also to the Adult Day Care Centers of Las Vegas and Henderson who had the patience to deal with Beecher's unusual disease. They had never had someone in their facility with FTD, let alone someone as young as Beecher. Most of the people that went there had Alzheimer's or other dementias and were much older. I'm sure it was a learning experience for them as well as me. And they handled things very well with him.

I'd like to personally thank the many caregivers at the different

Memory Care homes Beecher lived in. Thanks to Wendy and Alexa especially at Sterling Ridge who were there with him from day one. They helped make the transition from our home to his new home much more bearable. Also, thanks to Francesca, the Director of TLC (True Loving Care) and the many caregivers there, especially Diana who treated him with respect. She was the only one I felt Beecher completely trusted. She was always by his side and the only one who could physically help him up from the chair to a standing position by herself. To Myra and the other caregivers and to the patients who watched out for him, Dan, Miriam, Yum and Howard just to name a few, thank you.

And last but not least, a warm and loving thanks to Nathan Adelson Hospice, the social worker (Bridget), the nurse administrator (Kristie M), the case manager (Melinda), nurse in charge of meds (Kim), the chaplain (Dan Johnson), the nurses (Amy, Gayle and Lucy), and the Caseworker (Jerrie) who was right there even to the end. I can't give enough thanks for their roles in taking care of my husband at the end of his life. The countless hours they put in to make sure he had the best care possible and for the loving hugs and compassion, I will always be grateful.

To all these people who came into my life that I would not have had the pleasure of knowing, you were the best. Dantatsu! The best of the best! I honor you for helping me overcome my fears, for supporting us and mostly for your love and caring for my husband during the most difficult time of our lives.

I believe that caregiving is a state in which people become linked to one another through shared experiences which create a unique connection that results in comfort and a lifetime of memories.

Special thanks to everyone for the donations in lieu of flowers to theaftd.org honoring Beecher and the many donations from GoFundMe, GiveForward, and past customers of Beecher's and our friends. I often felt very humbled by the generosity of people. Many times, when I was having a bad day, I would go the mailbox and find a check for us. This act of kindness often brought me to my knees.

Someone once said "Death leaves a heartache no one can heal, but love leaves a memory no one can steal." I have 28 years of memories with Beecher, but I think I can breathe a little easier now. Life is a balance of holding on and letting go. I have to let go and find out who I am now. It's time to exhale and go forward!

*"Sometimes in life we just need a hug,
no words, no advice, just a hug to make you feel you matter."*

*Thanks to all of you for making us feel we matter!
Hugs to all of you for being a part of our lives.*

"TIME LIKE THE FUTURE"
BEECHER A. TRAIL | 8/17/96

Time like the future,
Runs on and on,
And it splits our souls,
Every day, until the day is done.

Thoughts just like words,
Create the deeds we do,
They shape our minds,
They make us blue.

Yet, change is near,
When we steer a path,
Be seeing clearly,
It's only truth that lasts.

It is not the darkest night,
But it is the morning sun,
That creates this journey,
Makes the metaphor the fun.

I don't know where I got the following message from, but I believe it's a message Beecher would have sent to me as it sounds like the words he would say to me:

While I must leave you for a little while, please do not grieve and shed wild tears and hug your sorrow to you through the years.

Instead, start out bravely with a gallant smile; and for my sake and in my name live on and do all the things the same. Feed not your loneliness on empty days, instead fill each waking hour in useful ways, reach out your hand in comfort and in cheer and I in turn will comfort you and hold you near; and never, never be afraid to die, for I am waiting for you in the sky!

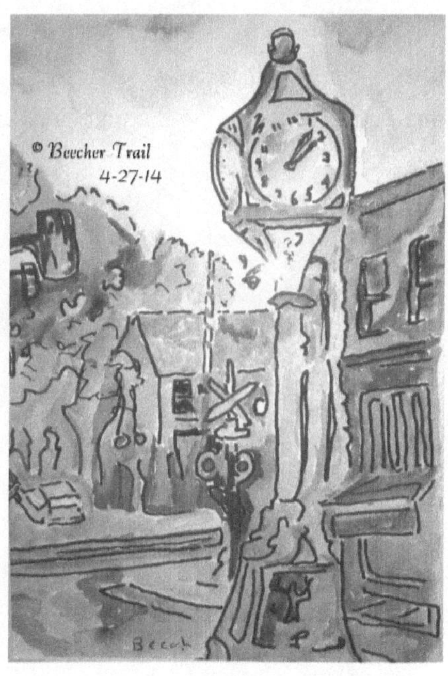

"Time"
Watercolor by Beecher Trail – 2014

"Time"
Time is just an inconvenience that separates us until love reaches
between our trembling fingers and draws us close together once again.

Beecher A. Trail
Written and given to Nancy in 1989

Creativity inspires ideas and ideas inspire change. Beecher's favorite
saying by Mahatma Gandhi says, "You must be the change you wish to
see in the world." I know that Beecher is watching over me and knows
that I am making that change, and I hope this book inspires changes in
the world and helps lead to a cure for FTD and other neurogenerative
diseases.

~Namaste~
(Namaste means showing a sign of respect)

www.ingramcontent.com/pod-product-compliance
Lightning Source LLC
Chambersburg PA
CBHW031527150726
47990CB00001B/81

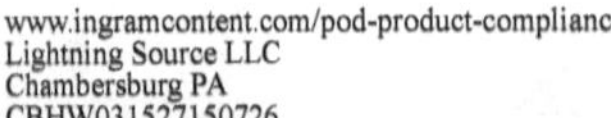